Chronic Disease Management in Primary Care

Quality and Outcomes

Edited by

Gill Wakley

Freelance General Practitioner
Visiting Professor
Centre for Health Policy and Practice
Staffordshire University

and

Ruth Chambers

General Practitioner
Clinical Dean
Staffordshire University
Head of Stoke-on-Trent Teaching PCT Programme

Radcliffe Publishing
Oxford • Seattle

Radcliffe Publishing Ltd
18 Marcham Road
Abingdon
Oxon OX14 1AA
United Kingdom

www.radcliffe-oxford.com
Electronic catalogue and worldwide online ordering facility.

British Library Cataloguing in Publication Data

Contents

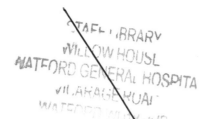

Preface

'Good chronic disease management can help to prevent crises and deterioration, and enable people living with chronic conditions to attain the best possible quality of life.'[1,2]

Up to three-quarters of people over 75 years are suffering from chronic disease, and this figure is rising. Around 45% of those with chronic disease suffer from more than one condition. Eighty per cent or so of consultations in general practice in the UK relate to chronic disease. People with more than one condition make much higher use of health care.

This book has been designed to help general practice teams improve their chronic disease management through problem-based learning (PBL). It focuses on the ten clinical fields for which there are quality indicators in the General Medical Services (GMS) contract as well as medicines management, and patient safety. The book helps you to understand how you can run PBL in-house in your practice. One of your practice team will need to facilitate the PBL sessions and to ensure that you plan the changes you decide are needed to improve your chronic disease management services.

The best and most cost-effective outcomes for patients in primary care are achieved when everyone involved works together, learns together, engages in clinical audit of outcomes together, and generates innovation to ensure progress in practice and service. Primary care team working leads to better detection, treatment, follow-up and outcomes for patients.

Teamworking can improve access to excellent care by freeing up highly qualified staff to do complex tasks and provide enhanced job satisfaction to those providing services. The team includes the patient and carer, and all those who work to provide services for their patients. The primary care team must link into the wider framework within your primary care organisation (PCO) and that of social care, secondary care, voluntary care and public health for effective chronic disease management – wherever you work in the UK.

Looking at ways of working better together

To explore how primary care teams might work together to solve problems and improve patient care, you can look at problem issues around the management of patient care that have occurred in your own practice. You might prefer to work through one or two of the examples outlined in each of the chapters and use it to guide you in a later discussion of one of your own problems. Add in any other points that occur in your discussions – the examples given are just an outline and not meant to be all inclusive! Sample checklists are included in each chapter that you might photocopy and use to identify who does what and when. If you feel that you have insufficient knowledge to guide you, use the summaries about clinical management in the second half of each chapter and follow up the references if you need to learn more. Then make your action plan and meet up again to review and evaluate progress matched to the quality and outcomes framework.[3]

References

1 Colin-Thomé D and Belfield G (2004) *Improving Chronic Disease Management*. Department of Health, London.

2 Department of Health (2004) *Chronic Disease Management: a compendium of information*. Department of Health, London.

3 General Practitioners Committee/The NHS Confederation (2003) *New GMS Contract. Investing in General Practice*. British Medical Association, London.

About the editors

Gill Wakley started in general practice in 1966, but transferred to community medicine shortly afterwards and then into public health. A desire for increased contact with patients caused a move back into general practice, together with community gynaecology. She has been combining the two, in varying amounts, ever since.

Throughout she has been heavily involved in learning and teaching. She was in a training general practice, became an instructing doctor and a regional assessor in family planning, and is a visiting professor at Staffordshire University. Like Ruth, she has run all types of educational initiatives and activities from individual mentoring and instruction, to small group work, plenary lectures, distance learning programmes, workshops, and courses for a wide range of health professionals and lay people.

Ruth Chambers has been a GP for more than 20 years and is currently the head of the Stoke-on-Trent Teaching Primary Care Trust programme and Clinical Dean at Staffordshire University. Ruth has worked with the Royal College of General Practitioners to enable GPs to gather evidence about their learning and standards of practice whilst striving to be *excellent* GPs. Ruth has co-authored a series of books with Gill designed to help readers draw up their own personal development plans or practice learning plans around key clinical topics.

About the contributors

Simon Ellis has been a consultant neurologist at the University Hospital of North Staffordshire for 10 years where he runs the neurovascular (TIA) clinic. He is a visiting professor in neurosciences at Staffordshire University. Simon has been involved in medical education, both undergraduate and graduate, for many years and runs appraisal training for medical educators. He has published on general neurology, appraisal and epilepsy.

Wendy Garcarz is an education and development specialist with a proven record of accomplishment in primary care. She has 20 years experience in education and training management in both the public and private sectors. Wendy has spent the last 10 years working in primary care, developing primary care clinicians and support workers in service commissioning, continuing professional development, strategic planning and service innovations. She is the chief executive of 4 health, an organisational development consultancy specialising in sustainable change through workforce investment. Wendy and her colleagues work with all types of healthcare organisations (wendy@4-health.biz).

Sarah Hands is a GP, senior lecturer at Staffordshire University, an appraiser and a former multidisciplinary educational lead for her local PCT. She has considerable experience in teaching across the disciplines on a variety of primary care related topics. Sarah has been influential in promoting inter-disciplinary education and workplace learning as part of locality schemes. Her key areas of interest are communication skills and practice based facilitated learning. Sarah has published papers on hearing loss in the elderly in general practice; educational evaluation of GPs' learning; and facilitation of the RCGP's Membership by Assessment of Performance.

Pat Hibberd is a principal lecturer for professional education in the Faculty of Health and Sciences at Staffordshire University, leading on the MSc Professional Education in Health Care. Her professional background is in nursing, midwifery and health visiting. Pat also works on secondment to the NHSU West Midlands as a learning coordinator for special projects and as part of this role is coordinating a collaborative project focusing on learning needs analysis in the context of the NHS Knowledge and Skills Framework (KSF).

Pete Osborne is a part-time pharmacist and full-time medical student. After graduating from Aston University and subsequently completing his pre-registration, Pete took a year to travel the world. Since his return he has worked as a community and primary care pharmacist before switching careers to retrain in medicine at Warwick University.

Alistair Pullan graduated from Aberdeen University in 1985. Having completed his pre-registration house jobs in Aberdeen and Inverness he moved to England, completing the North Staffordshire General Practitioner Vocational Training Scheme in 1990. Since then he has worked as a full-time principal in general practice in Stoke-on-Trent. He was awarded the Diploma in Practical Dermatology by the University of Wales College of Medicine in 2001. In addition to his work as a general practitioner, Alistair is a GP with Special Interest in dermatology.

Paul Roberts has been a GP principal since 1988. Currently he is clinical lead at a PCT practice in Stoke-on-Trent. He has a longstanding interest in palliative care and holds the diploma in palliative medicine from the University of Wales. Paul was clinical assistant at the Springhill Hospice in Rochdale and has a particular interest in developing systems for providing social care for patients with terminal illness and their families. He was primary care cancer lead for Rochdale and Middleton PCTs and helped to write the North West Cancer network primary care strategy. Paul can think of no particular reason why you should want to believe his text other than the general desire to humour a man with a chain saw and a manic cackle.

Andy Spooner is a full-time GP who acted for the NHS Confederation in negotiating the quality and outcomes framework of the GMS contract. His general practice underwent a change from reactive disease management to systematic care of illness. Andy has spent time investigating change management in many spheres and relating ideas to the real situation of a challenging practice environment.

Mark Waters is a full-time GP, husband and father of three, living and working in Hereford. He has spent the best part of a decade as a GP tutor, latterly at the local PCT setting up protected learning time for primary healthcare teams, and facilitating problem-based learning. Despite a vast range of educational work, Mark remains a full-time GP, and is actively involved in the practice, providing a GP with Special Interest dermatology service, doing all the nurse appraisals, and is the practice clinical governance and education lead. Mark has a Diploma in Medical Education and is currently engaged in research into GP trainer development for the Masters Award.

Acknowledgements

Shropshire and Staffordshire Health Authority commissioned the bulk of the material in this book as in-practice learning sessions, from a team at the Faculty of Health and Sciences at Staffordshire University. We are grateful to it for agreeing that the material can be published in book form.

1

Problem-based learning (PBL): how to do it

This chapter introduces you to the principles of problem-based learning (PBL). You will see how your primary healthcare team (PHCT) can use PBL to assist in improving chronic disease management in your practice. This includes practical ideas on how a PBL session should be run, what sort of outcomes you can expect and what pitfalls to avoid.

Why PBL is important

Problem-based learning was first developed in Canada, at McMaster University Medical School during the 1960s and has rapidly influenced medical and nursing education worldwide.[1] It encourages a move away from traditional didactic instruction to a more learner-centred approach to learning. It challenges you and the rest of your team to develop the ability to think critically, analyse problems, and find the most appropriate learning resources yourselves. As well as helping to address important learning relating to your work, PBL helps you to learn *how to learn*.

Problem-based learning is very enjoyable and will increase your motivation to change your clinical practice and behaviour.[2,3] This motivation is likely to be transferred into actual change, for instance in relation to prescription writing. Problem-based learning conforms to many of the principles that characterise effective adult learning, in that it:

- is linked to day-to-day practice
- is a group-based activity
- is flexible, and 'personalised' to your own situation
- reinforces learning, through review.

What is PBL?

In PBL the 'problem' is used as the stimulus for learning. In some ways this is the opposite of your previous experience, where you would be expected to already know something, and then to apply this knowledge to solve a test problem.

In PBL, the purpose of considering the problem presented is to allow discussion, and the identification of what is already known, and crucially, **what is not yet known**. The next step is to address the identified learning needs and share the new knowledge at a later meeting. Finally, the group considers how the new learning can be applied.

This sequence is described in Box 1.1.

Box 1.1:   Sequence of problem-based learning

1   Problem is presented to group
2   Group discusses the information
3   Group establishes agreed 'facts'
4   Group identifies what else it needs to know
5   Areas for learning are divided up within the group, and responsibility for carrying out the necessary learning and research is shared
6   Group meets again to review what has been learnt and how the learning can be used

---

The principles of PBL are.

- Problem scenarios do not test skills and knowledge.
- The problems are open-ended – there is no 'correct answer'. As new information is gathered and shared, the group develops an understanding of the problem and the learning.
- Different groups will identify different learning needs.
- The group solves the problem for itself.
- The group must decide for itself how it chooses to address the learning issues it has identified.
- The process is complete once the learning has been applied in practice. Ideally, these changes in practice can be audited to reinforce and check on the nature of their application.

How do you do it?[4–7]

Some preparation is needed. Ill-prepared attempts at PBL are likely to result in confusion and disappointment! The essential components are.

1   A group that is willing to learn together.
2   Someone to facilitate who understands the PBL process and can involve everyone in your team.
3   A PBL scenario that stimulates relevant discussion.

Planning checklist

Use the following checklist to help with your PBL planning.

Do you have time to do this?

A typical PBL session will take two to three hours to complete. You do not need to plough through a whole scenario if the team has identified enough learning issues to deal with earlier on in the case. The purpose of the PBL process is to engage your team in discussion, and to identify your collective learning needs. Then you can share, learn and plan for change.

Many practices will use protected learning time to carry out PBL so that all the team members can meet. Would this work for you? Does your primary care organisation (PCO) at least support you in this activity by for example providing emergency cover for the doctors, or could it? The time for PBL (like any other learning activity) needs to be properly protected – no ringing telephones, bleeps or other distractions!

Does everybody agree?

Most practice teams are complicated, diverse groups of people, who don't necessarily all want the same thing at the same time! So take time at a preliminary meeting for the lead facilitator to explain what PBL is about, and make sure everybody understands how it is expected to work. Provided that everyone in the team is happy to give it a go, a trial run often helps – as it is fun and engaging.

Who is going to be involved?

Problem-based learning works best when the group includes a full range of your primary healthcare team. Everyone brings their own perspective which is one of the strengths of the technique. Ideally, a PBL group includes doctors, nurses, healthcare assistants, practice manager, administrative and domestic staff, as well as attached staff such as social worker, pharmacist, health visitor, physiotherapist, podiatrist and midwife. Anyone who works in the team can be involved! And don't forget patients and their carers too.

Do you have a trained facilitator?

The facilitator should be familiar with techniques for running small groups successfully, as well as PBL principles. Is there someone in your team who can fulfil this role?

Is your group the right size?

Some people think the ideal group is around 8–12 people. However, PBL has been used successfully with groups slightly larger than this – up to 15. Anything larger and the group cannot function properly: some members of the group will not feel able to contribute, it will be difficult to hear what is being said, and there will be a tendency for the group to 'splinter' into smaller sections.

You could divide a larger group into two. You would then need two facilitators but the process will be much more effective and enjoyable. Both groups could use the same scenario and come together at the end to share their plans for learning.

Have you got the necessary equipment?

Each group will need a room large enough for everyone to sit in comfortably, without being disturbed. Get a flipchart, pens (that work!) and plenty of flipchart paper. Photocopy the problem case examples so that they can be handed out (one between two is probably enough) amongst the group members as you progress through the case. If you are facilitating watch the clock to pace the session.

Do you have a set of PBL scenarios?

This chapter includes a problem case example (*see* page 10) that you can use to get started, or you can turn to one of the other chapters. Further cases are available from other sources.[8]

... And remember:

PACE YOURSELVES!

Prioritise the learning issues identified to ensure that you are tackling a manageable number. It is better to address a small number of issues well, than to lose heart attempting too many at once.

Record your discussions, your action plan, resource requirements and expected outcomes. Think how you will collect evidence that demonstrates you have achieved what was planned. Use the form in Table 1.1 (*see* pages 7 and 8) to record these aspects of your PBL sessions, when you focus your session on your own real-life practice problem(s).

Running small groups

Three characteristics need to be present for small-group work.

1   Every member of the group should be an active participant. This is one very important way in which small group work differs from lectures, or large-group discussions. A small enough number of people are involved, and there is a facilitator to oversee the process as well as provide a balancing influence. A facilitator helps those who are reticent about contributing and restrains others who are more voluble so that all colleagues have a chance to contribute.
2   Have a specific task. Everyone should be aiming to achieve the same thing from the group work – otherwise it is unlikely that the group will be able to work as a unit.
3   The kind of learning that small groups can achieve goes deeper than just memorising lists of facts or procedures. It arises from people's experiences and therefore has much greater meaning – and benefits that are much longer lasting. Group members should be helped to think back over their own experiences and be prepared to share those with the rest of the group.

Being the facilitator

If you are the facilitator:

1 Before the group starts

Be prepared! Read through the preparatory paperwork, the scenario, the intended learning outcomes and this guide! Think about the time and space the group will be working in. Is the room comfortable? Are the chairs arranged so that everyone can see all the other group members? Do you know where the toilets are and what the scheduled start and finish times are? Arrive in plenty of time on the day so that you can feel in control.

2 Starting the group

You are now all in the room and sitting in the chairs you have carefully arranged. So what next? The first step is to allow the group to get to know and trust one another. The effectiveness of the group work will be helped enormously by spending a little time at the outset on 'ice-breaking'. This is relevant even when a PHCT is meeting together to learn. Not everyone will be familiar with all the people in the group and it is better to assume that introductions will be needed.

There are lots of ice-breaking games and techniques – you may have ones that you have experienced or used before.[9] There is no one 'right way'. Judge how much of an ice-breaker your group needs. If you are uncertain about what to do you could:

- **Start with a round of introductions**. Everyone in the group states their name, where they work, and something a bit more personal about themselves, in turn. This should be non-threatening and allow each person to offer something of themselves to the group. You could go first in a round like this to show what you are looking for from everyone else. Allow about two minutes per person for this bit.
- **Make a note of their names** (mentally, or on a piece of paper) as the members introduce themselves.
- **Have another exercise** –'What I am hoping to achieve from today's meeting' once the initial round is complete. Start with someone else in the group. Try to invite each person to speak using their name and thank them for their contribution before moving on to the next person. This demonstrates the kind of communication expected from group members, serves to reinforce your recall of people's names and helps to ensure that there is a shared agenda for the group.

3 Group rules

Explain how you expect people to behave so that it is easier to deal with unhelpful behaviour later (if it occurs!). Ask the group members to suggest 'ways of working' they would find helpful. Put the rules up on a flipchart as they are stated, and then display that flipchart sheet on the wall with Blu-tak so that they can be referred to again if necessary. Typical rules include:

- confidentiality
- mutual respect
- only one person talking at a time
- everyone needs to be involved.

4 Set the task

OK, so the group is now rolling – everyone knows each other, at least a bit, and they have a shared idea of why they have all come and how they will work together. Now, down to work!

5 Facilitate

As the discussion gets going, be prepared to allow it to flow – you may not need to intervene or contribute very much yourself. At some stage, though, there are several types of facilitation that could be required. Broadly speaking, the interventions you make will be directed either to the **task** of the group, or to **group maintenance**.

Ensure everyone is contributing. If you feel someone needs to be 'brought in' to the discussion, it might be appropriate to ask them specifically for an opinion, using their name: 'John – what do you think about that?', or more generally, if several group members are left out: 'What does everyone else think about that?'.

Steer the discussion back to the subject if it has wandered too far away from the point. But be careful because you do not want to stifle the flow. If the discussion seems to have gone off on a tangent, share this feeling with the group: 'I wonder if we have strayed away from our purpose here?'. You may find that the group readily agrees, and gets back on track. Alternatively, the group may be finding the discussion really helpful and wish to continue with it. You will then need to negotiate with the members: remind them of the objectives you had all agreed at the beginning, and get them to decide whether they want to abandon these and follow the new direction or return to the original plan. There is a tension here between leading the group to achieve the stated objectives of the meeting, or allowing the group to define its own purpose. Use your gut instinct.

Clarify contributions. Sometimes it will be helpful to explore a statement a little more deeply in a non-confrontational way: 'That sounds really interesting, Sheila – can you tell us a bit more about it?'. Summarise the discussion. A successful way of moving the discussion on is to summarise to the group what has been said so far. Do this in an exploratory way: 'Shall I try and summarise what we have agreed?' and check that members of the group agree with your version: 'Does that sound right to you all?'

Gain agreement before moving on to the next part of the scenario: 'Shall we move on to the next stage?'.

6 Ending the session

Let the group know that they are reaching the end of the available time: 'Can I just let you know that we will need to break for lunch in about ten minutes?'. This will also help you to close the discussion and draw conclusions.

Offer a debriefing at the end of the session. Allow enough time for this (in a session lasting 90 minutes, at least five minutes will be needed): 'Can we just summarise what we have learned from this?'.

7 Evaluation

Distribute a formal evaluation sheet at the end of the whole session. But informally evaluate the work of the group at the end of the session as well. Aim to do this with around five minutes to go. Make it clear that the work has been completed, thank the group for its work, and ask for comments from anyone in the group: 'Well, I'm afraid that's all we are going to have time for. Thank you everyone for working so hard. Has this session been useful for you?'. If time allows, you can ask for more detailed evaluation: 'What was most useful about this group session? What would you have liked to have done differently?'. Check that the initial objectives have been met.

Table 1.1 Recording form: problem-based learning discussion and action taken

Problem Case:

(*Write your own problem case here*)

Who do you need in your team?

Where you are now

Continued

What you do next

What extra resources might this require?

The outcomes

How would you demonstrate that you have achieved your outcomes?

What will the outcomes be?

The outcomes of PBL should be seen in two stages. In the first session you should involve everyone who can contribute to unpicking the problem, who has a contribution to make in devising the solutions. The second session might involve those who have taken on roles or responsibilities for action (*see* Table 1.2 on page 11 for example). It might be run as a feedback and review of progress on your action plan at the start of the next PBL session. Then you might move on to another clinical field and start again. The people attending each PBL session will probably vary, because of prior commitments, holidays, absence due to sickness, etc.

After the first session

The team will have met together and spent time discussing issues relevant to the work of the practice. Some scenarios will be clinical, others entirely non-clinical (such as issues around communication or appointment systems). The clinical scenarios will obviously benefit from the input of non-clinical members of the team too.

The discussion will have helped everyone to develop a shared understanding of the way patient care is provided. Some assumptions will have been challenged, some knowledge shared, and your group will have identified a list of the most important issues that need to be learnt about next. You should prioritise these with an eye on what is possible in the real world. You can be confident that these learning needs are relevant, because the primary healthcare team have generated them through discussion of realistic scenarios.

By the end of the first session, members of the team will have agreed to take responsibility for addressing the various learning issues within an agreed timescale. This might involve researching some facts (such as specific drug interactions, or the effectiveness of some lifestyle modification in hypertension management), or involve working in collaboration with other members of the team to produce a protocol, or carry out an audit. Document these learning issues and agreed timescales.

After the second session

The second session might be a month after the first, or longer – it depends on what will work in your situation and what you have all agreed to do. You should review the learning issues from last time and share the work done by group members since the last session. Often there will be suggestions for changes in practice. Discuss these in a realistic way and try to reach a consensus. Make plans for auditing changes in practice at this stage too. Recording progress means that you are monitoring the learning – so things should not get missed. Communicate all suggestions and changes to the rest of the practice team.

Evaluation

It is vital to evaluate the effectiveness of any educational activity. Then you will be reviewing that the intended outcomes are being achieved, and exploring ways that a similar session can be made more effective next time.

What are the pitfalls of PBL groups?

Problem-based learning requires a properly functioning group, and a facilitator who understands the process of group facilitation and of PBL. The group process is helped by good facilitation – but some practice teams will not be well suited to the PBL approach. Perhaps there is poor communication within the team, politically motivated positions, over-emphasis on hierarchy within the team or even sabotage from some members of the team. Ensuring agreement and understanding about the process of the PBL session at the outset can minimise this problem, but sometimes difficulties can still arise when carrying out group-based learning.

Another possible drawback of the PBL process is that learning can be a little unstructured. This does not matter to everyone, but some people find learning more effective if they can see the structure at the outset. If most people are like this in your team then PBL may not be for you. It will help to share notes of your action planning and news of progress made.

Don't forget that PBL is only an *option*. No one method of learning is a panacea – and it is important to be prepared to vary the learning techniques you use.

An example of a PBL scenario: type 1 diabetes mellitus

The problem case example that follows about a patient with type 1 diabetes has been worked through in some detail. A list of learning issues that *could* result from a discussion appears throughout the sequence of this scenario. Of course, what you discuss and learn is dependent on the members of your group, their situations and the facilitator. The problem case example is typical of the kind of scenario used for PBL in primary healthcare teams.

Appoint someone from the group to be the 'scribe' – to stand by the flipchart, ready to write down important facts and learning issues as they arise. You could divide the flipchart sheet into two halves down the middle with important facts on one side and learning issues on the opposite side to make this clearer.

If you are the facilitator, take the stages one at a time and ask someone in the group to read through each new section. After the section has been read, ask the group an open question such as: 'Any comments?'. Allow the discussion to flow. As people mention items ask the scribe to note them down. If the group identifies something it is not sure about, clarify with it that this is the case: 'this sounds like a learning need for us all – shall we note it down?'. Look at the list of expected learning issues as you progress. If something has not been discussed, you could ask an open question about that subject, if you wish. Move on to the next stage when you and the group feel ready. It will probably take you at least two hours to work through the nine stages, and you may not get that far in the time you allot to a single PBL session.

With about 15 minutes of your allotted time left, ask the group to spend some time looking at the identified learning issues. Which are the most important priorities? Of these, which ones can you and others in the team realistically tackle in time for the next session? Who is going to take responsibility for addressing each one?

Give a copy of Table 1.2 to everyone taking part and use it to stimulate thought at the start of the session or as a checklist at the end.

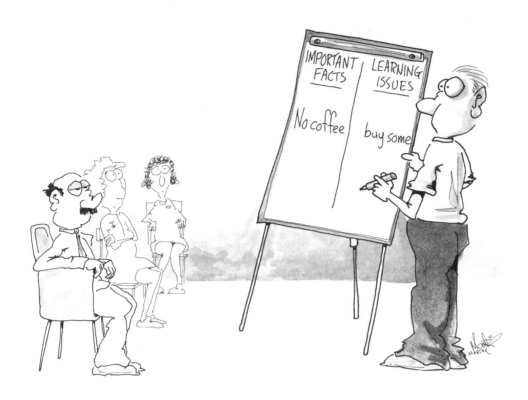

Problem case example

Who do you need in your team?

The team of the Shire Practice working on this PBL session includes:

Dr Andy Williams
Dr Duncan Blue
Dr Kenny Evertrue
Dr Sheila Bow
Sister Goodbody
Sister Goodhead
Sister Goodspirit
Mrs Alison Shipp, practice manager
Mrs Kerry Counter, receptionist
Miss Jen Type, secretary
Mr Jim Keen, pharmacist.

Table 1.2: Role and responsibilities checklist – *for each task tick the box for each team member who has a role or responsibility – then note your role and responsibilities for the task*

Completed by: *Mrs Kerry Counter, receptionist*

Task	Doctor	Practice nurse	District nurse	Receptionist	Practice manager	Practice secretary	Other	What are your roles and your responsibilities?
Identifying patients who might have chronic disease								
Recording diagnosis of a chronic disease within the practice	✔	✔		✔	✔	✔		*e.g. Admin. side is done properly; up-to-date referral folder in every consulting area; faxing/telephoning and recording referrals when done; reminding locum about system if needed*
Managing complications of treatment								
Practice-specific one								
Practice-specific two								

Stage 1

Problem Case:

Harry Bull is a 19-year-old patient at the Shire practice. His family is well known to the practice team, although they have been pretty fit and well over the years. Harry did very well in his A-levels, and has a place to go to University next September. He has been travelling, but has returned from Southern Italy because he has been feeling less well. He comes to see Dr Evertrue in an evening appointment the day after he gets home.

He describes a 10-day illness with the following symptoms.

- Tiredness
- Slight nausea
- Increased frequency of urination
- Being more thirsty, but has put this down to the hot climate in Italy.

Dr Evertrue wonders if he might have a urine infection, or possibly just a virus. He considers the possibility of diabetes. He arranges for a blood specimen to check his full blood count, urea and electrolytes and random glucose. Sister Goodbody has left for the evening, so the receptionist books an appointment for Harry for first thing in the morning.

GROUP DISCUSSION

Box 1.2: Potential learning issues

- Symptoms of type 1 diabetes
- Appropriate urgency for handling a possible new case of diabetes
- Organisation of care in the practice – who takes blood tests? What happens at the end of the day when something unusual presents?
- Communication within the PHCT
- Safety netting

Stage 2

Problem Case continued

Later that evening, Harry feels less well. He has developed abdominal pain, generalised aches and pains and a headache. His mother realises that he is ill and calls the out-of-hours service. He is given an appointment at the primary care centre 90 minutes later. Sixty minutes later, he has become even more unwell, with rapid breathing. His mother calls an ambulance, and he is taken to A&E, where he is diagnosed with diabetic ketoacidosis, and treated in the usual way.

GROUP DISCUSSION

Box 1.3:   Potential learning issues

- Principles of management of diabetic ketoacidosis. What should be done in primary care?
- Organisation of out-of-hours care

Stage 3

Problem Case continued

The following week, Harry is discharged from hospital. He has type 1 diabetes and has been started on an insulin regimen:

8am: 16 units Isophane
              8 units Soluble
7pm: 8 units Isophane
              4 units Soluble

He has seen the diabetes nurse specialist and has been given her telephone number to call if necessary. The surgery has received a handwritten carbon-copy discharge note with this information on, although some of the writing is hard to read. He has an outpatient appointment in the diabetic clinic in six weeks' time. The letter is addressed to Dr Blue, who is Harry's registered GP. He is surprised to receive it as he was not aware that Harry had come back from his gap-year travels. In the Shire Practice, Dr Williams and Sister Goodspirit see all the patients with diabetes. Dr Blue puts the letter in Dr Williams' post.

Box 1.4: Potential learning issues

- Insulin regimens
- Role of diabetic nurse specialists
- Quality of discharge information from the hospital
- Shared lists and personal lists in general practice
- Organisation of diabetic care in practice

Stage 4

Problem Case continued

Two days later, Harry's mother calls the diabetic nurse specialist (DNS) concerned about how Harry is coping. He seems withdrawn and angry and has recurrent headaches. He does not want to keep measuring his blood sugar and thinks that a mistake has been made in his diagnosis – and has missed some of his insulin injections. The DNS is away on a course. A message is left for the duty doctor at the surgery – Dr Blue as it happens, that day.

Dr Blue decides it would be best to visit Harry and does so that afternoon. On his way round Dr Blue feels quite anxious because he is not sure about the details of insulin treatment and hopes he won't be asked too many technical questions. He wishes that the hospital team could provide more comprehensive cover. If it takes everything over and GPs get de-skilled, it's not good passing the problems back whenever it suits it, he thinks.

Box 1.5: Potential learning issues

- The patient's emotional reaction to diagnosis and adjustment
- De-skilling of health professionals
- Are findings from hospital letters entered into the patient's computer record?
- Systems for recording and actioning changes to treatment

Stage 5

Problem Case continued

When Dr Blue visits, he finds that Harry is in a low mood, and having a lot of difficulty adjusting to the idea that he has diabetes. Harry wants to know.

- Why has this happened to him?
- Will he always have to inject himself twice a day?
- How long will it be before he is able to drink alcohol again?
- Will he have to delay going up to University?

Dr Blue deals with the questions as best he can – but has to admit that he is not an expert. He encourages Harry to contact the hospital DNS tomorrow, and arrange another meeting with her. He emphasises how important it is to use the insulin regularly, as directed.

Before evening surgery he chats to Dr Williams about the visit. Dr Williams is interested, and supportive. He asks Dr Blue 'did you let him know about contacting the Driver and Vehicle Licensing Agency (DVLA)?'.

GROUP DISCUSSION

Box 1.6: Potential learning issues

- Aetiology of type 1 diabetes
- Lifestyle advice in type 1 diabetes
- Informing the DVLA
- Housebound patients – who takes the lead: community nurses, nurse practitioners, GPs, secondary care?

Stage 6

Problem Case continued

Time passes and six months later Harry has been stabilised on insulin glargine for the previous three months. In fact he felt so well he started getting back into the social scene again and driving his car.

Unfortunately he has had a road traffic accident. The circumstances are not clear, as he was alone in the car. He has a fractured pelvis and a fractured left radius.

Before he is properly up and about, he is due for a diabetic check at the hospital. He cannot easily get there, and his mother rings the surgery to ask if 'one of the nurses can come and do the diabetic check?'.

Box 1.7:   Potential learning issues

- New insulin regimens (insulin pumps?)
- Appropriate training for tasks – who should carry out diabetic checks?
- Hypoglycaemia in people with type 1 diabetes

Stage 7

Problem Case continued

A receptionist leaves a message in the district nurse's book for the following day. One of the community nursing team carries out the diabetic check on Harry. She checks his blood pressure and weight, looks at his record of blood glucose readings (taken using a glucose meter he was given by a friend) and tells him he is doing very well.

Box 1.8:   Potential learning issues

- Recording of information on computer when gathered by community staff – does it happen?
- Calibration of glucometers or understanding how to use them correctly

---

Stage 8

Problem Case continued

The following year Dr Bow is carrying out an audit with Mrs Shipp looking at the performance indicators for diabetes in the quality and outcomes framework. Any patients with diabetes who do not have an adequate record are written to and asked to make an appointment to see Sister Goodspirit.

Amongst those with poor records is Harry Bull. Missing information includes.

- Fundoscopy/retinal screening
- Peripheral pulses
- Foot examination
- No 'flu vaccination
- Microalbuminuria screening.

He is not the only one. In many cases the patients have been seen at a hospital clinic, but the letters do not give details of what kind of diabetic checks have been carried out. Dr Bow decides to raise this at the next practice meeting.

Box 1.9:   Potential learning issues

- Quality and outcomes framework
- Standards of care in primary and secondary care. Are we all working to the same protocols?
- 'Flu vaccination in people with diabetes
- Transferring information from hospital letters into general practice records – what systems are needed?

Stage 9

Problem Case continued

Harry receives a letter inviting him to a review appointment with Sister Goodspirit. He is not keen to attend. He feels he is getting plenty of input from the hospital clinic – and anyway he feels he understands his condition well now, and wants to have more independence in making management decisions. He does not make an appointment.

Box 1.10:   Potential learning issues

- Self-monitoring in people with type 1 diabetes: who controls management decisions?
- Co-ordination of care between hospital and primary care – does it work?

And finally

With about 15 minutes of your allotted time left, ask the group to spend some time looking at the learning issues you have identified as you have worked through the nine stages. Then:

- decide together which are the most important priorities. Some of these priorities will involve individual members of the team learning more about the clinical topic, some will involve learning and practising new skills, some will mean members of the team changing the way they work and having new responsibilities. You will be discussing how to improve the way you deliver services as a team, how to revise your clinical protocols and enable GPs and staff to adhere to them, when and how you should be undertaking clinical audit, how to improve communication between team members and with patients, and those working in hospital, etc

- make an action plan, specifying who is going to take responsibility for addressing each priority area, including who is responsible for the progress and completion of the action plan
- fix a date for your next review meeting
- agree which priorities can be realistically tackled by the review meeting
- check progress at the review meeting and thereafter continue to revisit and monitor the action plan.

References

1   Barrows H (1986) A taxonomy of problem-based learning methods. *Medical Education.* **20**: 481–6.

2   Zeitz HJ (1999) Problem based learning: development of a new strategy for effective continuing medical education. *Allergy and Asthma Proceedings.* **20(5)**: 317–21.

3   Hughes L and Lucas J (1997) An evaluation of problem-based learning in the multi-professional education curriculum for the health professions. *Journal of Interprofessional Care.* **11**: 77–88.

4   Parsell G and Bligh J (1998) Interprofessional learning. *Postgraduate Medical Journal.* **74**: 89–95.

5   Kilminster S, Hale C, Lascelles M *et al.* (2004) Learning for real life: patient-focused inter-professional workshops offer added value. *Medical Education.* **38(7)**: 717–26.

6   Rushmer R, Kelly D, Lough M *et al.* (2004) Introducing the Learning Practice – I. The characteristics of learning. *Journal of Evaluation in Clinical Practice.* **10(3)**: 375–86.

7   Wilcock PM, Campion Smith C and Head M (2002) The Dorset Seedcorn Project: interprofessional learning and continuous quality improvement in primary care. *British Journal of General Practice.* **52(Suppl)**: S39–44.

8   O'Brien D and Downey PF (1999) *Problem-Based Learning for the Primary Health Care Team: facilitators' pack.* John Ross Postgraduate Centre, Hereford.

9   Chambers R, Wakley G, Iqbal Z *et al.* (2002) *Prescription for Learning: techniques, games and activities.* Radcliffe Medical Press, Oxford.

2

Team-based learning

Why team-based learning is important

Primary care is delivered in teams in the UK. Some practice teams are well established with members all working under one roof and holding regular meetings. In other cases the team is more diffuse – with attached staff sharing the care of patients with GPs and practice nurses, and administrative staff in the surgery building providing linking and co-ordinating roles.

Inter-professional boundaries are less clear these days. It can be difficult to be sure who is the lead professional in an individual patient's care at any given time. Is it the GP, the community nurse or the practice nurse?

Different professionals have overlapping skills and knowledge.[1] We work as part of a team because our combined, complementary strengths deliver broad-based, effective care to our patients. Teams of organised, caring, well-trained administrative staff enable clinicians to get on with the clinical tasks, as well as providing their own contributions to the well-being of patients.

Discussion in groups helps you to see new perspectives on your problems, and take pride in helping others along the way. Organising learning in teams makes provision of protected time easier.

The Bristol Children's Heart Surgery enquiry[2] and the Victoria Climbié enquiry[3] urged more collaborative learning, across the traditional divides between professional groups.[4] It is not what people have in common, but their differences that can create a dynamic environment for successful team working and learning.[5]

The GMS contract recognises the importance of team-based learning. Quality and outcomes framework points are awarded in relation to working with colleagues.[6] Multidisciplinary working in the delivery of the expected quality framework is valued. Some of the education and training quality indicators are shown in Table 2.1.

Why inter-professional learning is important

Inter-professional learning has all the benefits of learning in teams, with additional advantage coming from the mixture of individuals involved, particularly in enhancing communication skills between professionals.[7]

Where inter-professional learning happens regularly there is more likely to be a learning organisation culture.[8,9] Successful learning teams are not born, they are created, and then carefully nurtured![10]

Table 2.1:   Quality and outcomes measures for education and training[6]

Criteria	Indicator	Points
Education 2	The practice has undertaken a minimum of six significant event reviews in the past three years. Each report to consist of short commentary setting out relevant history, circumstances of the episode and an analysis of conclusions drawn. Evidence of clinical and organisational changes resulting from the analysis of these cases	4
Education 6	The practice conducts annual review of patients' complaints and suggestions to ascertain general learning points that are shared with the team. Reports or minutes of team meetings where learning points discussed, with note of the changes made as a result	3
Education 7	The practice has undertaken a minimum of 12 significant event reviews in past three years, which include (if these have occurred): • any death occurring in the practice premises • two new cancer diagnoses • two deaths where terminal care has taken place at home • one patient complaint • one suicide • one Section under the Mental Health Act Each case report must consist of a short commentary setting out relevant history, circumstances of episode and an analysis of the conclusions drawn. Evidence of clinical and organisational changes resulting from analysis of these cases	4

Multidisciplinary learning is not necessarily inter-professional learning.[4]

• Multidisciplinary education describes a situation where different professional groups learn *alongside* each other.
• Inter-professional education is where different professional groups learn *with*, *from* and *about* each other. There is an opportunity to learn about other members of the team through interaction, discussion, and problem solving, as well as developing specific new skills and knowledge to support patient care.

Inter-professional learning is the basis upon which a practice professional development plan[11] (PPDP) is built. This plan should incorporate the developmental aspirations of the whole practice team, taking into consideration national NHS priorities, local PCO targets, and the health needs of the practice population. It will also include plans for learning from audit, complaints and significant event analyses. It records the way the practice team has worked together to identify what needs to be done and the learning that will be needed to support practice development. All members of the practice team must be contributing for this to be a valid and meaningful process, as well as supporting each other with a proper understanding of each other's roles.

Understanding more about each other

Understanding and respecting each other's situation and background is key to facilitating the working together of primary care team members from different professional groups. You should be aware of the different pathways of education, training and continuing certification that different professionals follow.[12]

How to generate a programme of team-based learning

Who should be involved?

The most effective team-based, inter-professional learning involves a wide mix of the people who work in the primary healthcare team. This could typically include doctors, practice nurses, receptionists, practice manager, dispenser or pharmacist, health visitors, community nurses, social workers, midwives, occupational therapists and podiatrists.

Organising the learning

There is a logical flow to the organisation of the learning, which loops back on itself (*see* Figure 2.1).

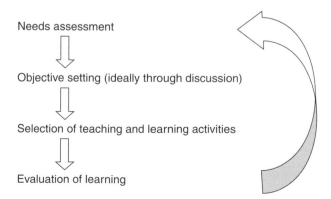

Needs assessment

Objective setting (ideally through discussion)

Selection of teaching and learning activities

Evaluation of learning

Figure 2.1: Flow diagram illustrating the organisation of learning.

Setting aims and objectives for learning

Turn learning needs into objectives. So far, you have considered *why* it is a good idea to learn in teams, and in Chapter 3 you will discover how you can identify *what to* learn about. This section focuses on *how* you can organise the learning.

Formulate the aim, a global expression of your intentions when organising any educational activity. Your aim may be quite broad – for example with diabetes: 'To improve the management and care of patients with diabetes'.

This aim identifies the subject being covered on a given day, but does not help much if you want to prepare for the session, or if you want to be able to measure how successful the session has been at the end. For this, setting *objectives* helps more. These are much more specific statements that describe what you hope to learn by the end of your PBL session. For example, by the end of the session, you will be able to:

- list the different kinds of diabetes
- identify who has responsibility for the on-going management of patients with diabetes within the team
- produce a protocol for the management of an unconscious patient with diabetes
- list the performance indicators for diabetes in the quality and outcomes framework
- understand the current diagnostic criteria for type 2 diabetes
- describe the initial management of a patient presenting with type 2 diabetes

... and so on.

Involve the team in setting the objectives. The educational session will then have more meaning and relevance for it. This works best when the team sets its objectives soon after it has identified its learning needs. Once the learning needs are identified, the group can split up according to anticipated team roles, and consider what it would like to achieve from addressing its learning needs. Remember the SMART acronym when setting objectives. This describes the characteristics of an objective, as:

- **S**pecific
- **M**easurable
- **A**chievable
- **R**elevant
- **T**imescale.

To illustrate this with the focused set of objectives given above.

- **Specific**: list the different kinds of diabetes.
- **Measurable**: each team member could fill in a form at the end, which could include the prompt 'list the different kinds of diabetes'.
- **Achievable**: the session will cover type 1 and type 2 diabetes.
- **Relevant**: clinicians will plan different kinds of management for diabetes and administrative staff will have a basic understanding of the classification of diabetes.
- **Timescale**: 'by the end of the session we will ...'.

Not all learning can be planned of course, and learning outcomes also include the informal learning that each member of the team takes away. Some of this learning may occur during coffee time, some of it will happen as a result of a person's train of thought going off at a tangent in the middle of a session. Some learning may suddenly 'click' on the journey home.

Selecting teaching and learning methods for your team

Variety is the key. If team-based learning sessions are all run the same way, they will start to feel staid and predictable.[13] Try to make your selection of teaching and learning activities appropriate to the kind of learning needs and objectives your team has. If one or more of the objectives relates to a protocol for use by the team for instance, then involve all team members in discussing the draft protocol as one of your learning activities.[14,15] Consider whether the following methods might suit your learning objectives and the dynamics of the team.[12]

- Problem-based learning scenarios. You might do these in-house after a practice needs assessment or at a PCO-wide educational half-day.
- Undertaking needs assessment activities themselves provide opportunities for learning, such as a significant event review discussion or 360 degree appraisal of team members.
- Inter-practice visiting gives you a chance to review other people's working patterns and exchange ideas of how to do it.

Evaluating your learning activity

You want to know whether team-based learning has been successful. Evaluation occurs after you have identified relevant learning and service development needs, clarified your objectives and subsequently selected and undertaken appropriate teaching and learning activities. It often leads to the identification of further learning and service development needs, so that the circle, or upwards spiral, of development continues.

Evaluation might be simple verbal feedback of what individuals thought went well or less well at the learning session. A more formal written evaluation will help you to plan and make changes for next time. Possible questions to ask on your evaluation form include the following.

- Was the aim of the session clear to you at the beginning?
- List three things that you have learned during the session.
- What changes to the session would you make if we were running it another time?
- How will your practice change after the PBL session?
- Please describe what you have enjoyed, and what you feel worked less well in the session.
- Did you have the opportunity to contribute today?

Free-hand comments are particularly valuable in evaluating whether those participating enjoyed the session and felt that they had benefited. Other more complex methods can be used.[16,17]

How to run team-based learning sessions

The following is a list of helpful hints for running a team-based learning session. The hints are the same as those for PBL.

- **Prepare for the sessions**: to get the best out of each learning session you need to prepare well (*see* page 2).
- **Establish trust**: decide upon group rules at an early stage (see page 5).
- **Warm up exercises**: create an environment conducive to interactive learning. Introductory exercises are a good way of getting the team off to a flying start.
- **Maintain a good learning environment**: this is essential for any successful learning interaction to ensure that everyone takes part and is interested and motivated.[18,19] Basically:
  - Provide a warm supportive setting with a relaxed atmosphere – protected time for learning with no mobile phones or other interruptions.
  - Be nurturing, supportive and interested in participants' welfare – ensure individuals are comfortable and time is built in for refreshment breaks.
  - Cultivate a positive atmosphere and good interpersonal relationships between participants – to some extent this will depend upon the history of the team but much can be done during the course of a learning session to promote this.
  - Encourage everyone to engage in open discussion – they will own what is going on and this is more likely to result in effective learning.
  - Include suitable challenges appropriate to the needs of individuals in the team – with appropriate learning methods.
  - Material used by the team should be relevant to their roles – now or in the future. It should be practice based and not focused entirely on secondary care or PCO priority issues. If it is relevant for all the team then everyone can join in the learning process.
  - Be enthusiastic and motivate your colleagues to learn – a good facilitator can inspire even the most reluctant individual.
  - Promote self-confidence. Different professions learning together in a team can feel awkward at the outset. Each team member should feel that his or her contribution is valuable.
  - Encourage individual team members to identify and address their own learning needs.
  - Use a problem-based approach that allows team members to employ their problem-solving skills.

References

1 Parsell G and Bligh J (1998) Interprofessional learning. *Postgraduate Medical Journal*. **74**: 89–95.

2 Smith R (2001) One Bristol, but there could have been many. *BMJ*. **323**: 179–80.

3 Hall D (2003) Child protection – lessons from Victoria Climbié Enquiry. *BMJ*. **326**: 293–4.

4 Humphris D and Hean S (2004) Educating the future workforce: building the evidence about interprofessional learning. *Journal of Health Service Research and Policy*. **1**: 24–7.

5   Davies C (2000) Getting health professionals to work together. *BMJ*. **320**: 1021–2.

6   General Practitioners Committee/The NHS Confederation (2003) *New GMS Contract. Investing in General Practice*. GPC/NHS Confederation, London. www.nhsconfed.org/docs/annex_a_quality_indicators.doc

7   Kilminster S, Hale C, Lascelles M *et al.* (2004) Learning for real life: patient-focused interprofessional workshops offer added value. *Medical Education*. **38(7)**: 717–26.

8   Rushmer R, Kelly D, Lough M *et al.* (2004) Introducing the Learning Practice – I. The characteristics of learning. *Journal of Evaluation in Clinical Practice*. **10(3)**: 375–86.

9   Wilcock PM, Campion Smith C and Head M (2002) The Dorset Seedcorn Project: interprofessional learning and continuous quality improvement in primary care. *British Journal of General Practice*. **52(Suppl)**: S39–44.

10   McNair R, Brown R, Stone N *et al.* (2001) Rural interprofessional education: promoting teamwork in primary health. *Australian Journal of Rural Health*. **9(1)**: S19–26.

11   Chief Medical Officer (1998) *A Review of Continuing Professional Development in General Practice*. Department of Health, London.

12   Hands S and Hughes M (2003) *Educators Handbook*. National Association of Primary Care Educators UK, London.

13   Biggs J (2003) *Teaching for Quality Learning at University: what the student does* (2e). Society for Research into Higher Education, Buckingham.

14   Mohanna K, Wall D and Chambers R (2004) *Teaching Made Easy: a manual for health professionals* (2e). Radcliffe Publishing, Oxford.

15   Chambers R, Wakley G, Iqbal Z *et al.* (2002) *Prescription for Learning: techniques, games and activities*. Radcliffe Medical Press, Oxford.

16   Grant J, Evans K, May R *et al.* (1993) *An Evaluation Pack for Education in General Practice*. Joint Centre for Education in Medicine, London.

17   Fleming W (1998) *The Observation of Educational Events*. ASME, Edinburgh.

18   Harth SC, Bavanandan S, Thomas KE *et al.* (1992) The quality of student–tutor interactions in the clinical learning environment. *Medical Education*. **26**: 321–6.

19   Moore West M, Harrington DL, Mennin SP *et al.* (1986) Distress and attitudes toward the learning environment: effects of a curriculum innovation. *Proceedings of the Annual Conference on Research in Medical Education*. **25**: 293–300.

3

Assessing your learning and service development needs: effective chronic disease management

Introduction

Identify your learning needs as follows.

- Focus on your current performance as a practice team and spot any gaps. This helps to identify which particular chronic disease areas or aspect of practice management should be tackled first.
- Help everyone to reflect on their own role and performance. Help individuals to identify their personal learning needs in relation to their work with patients and the practice as a whole.
- Look at whether you are ready, as a practice, to make changes.

Review a case (or cases) with which your team has been involved to explore how your primary care team might work together to identify its learning needs and improve patient care. You may prefer to use the two example cases at the start of this chapter or read through them quickly before working on your own practice needs assessment based on your own problem case, using the Table on page 31. Include in your team people who will join in the problem-based learning discussion and be part of the solutions.

If you feel that you have insufficient knowledge to guide you in completing the problem-based learning, use the summary about needs assessment in the second part of this chapter (*see* page 37) and follow up the references if you need to learn more.

Example problem case 1

Problem Case:

An away day is organised for the practice to make plans for the future. It is agreed that there should be a small bonus payment to each member of staff for each extra 20 quality and outcomes points the practice achieves over the 750 points estimated by the primary care organisation. It emerges that nobody at the meeting, except the practice manager and senior partner, are sure what measurements and recording the quality and outcomes framework includes.

Who do you need in your team?

You might want a team that includes:

Reception staff
Practice manager
Clerical and secretarial staff
Practice nurses
Healthcare assistants (HCAs)
Doctors
Patients.

Where you are now

The doctors and practice nurses have just begun to get to grips with recording data for the areas for which they are responsible, e.g. the asthma and diabetes clinics. Most of the rest of the staff have almost no knowledge.

What you do next

This might include.

- Looking at the various areas in the quality and outcomes framework together and identifying two areas to work on.
- Allocating particular items to small groups of relevant staff who will:
  – identify what they need to learn about, e.g. being able to offer an appointment with a health professional within 24 hours, or aspects of medicines management
  – draw up a learning plan of the relevant areas
  – gather information
  – make an action plan together with the people affected, including patients
  – include everyone affected in planning change(s) needed
  – implement change(s)
  – evaluate the outcomes.
- Completing Table 3.1.

What extra resources might this require?

- Time for staff to identify and learn about relevant tasks.
- Time to make the action plan and ask patients what they need.
- Resources and support to make change(s).
- Time and expertise to evaluate change(s) made.
- Investment in new technology such as new telephone system, or different ways of working with an existing system.
- New computer stations or relocation of existing ones with new points of connection.

The outcomes

The outcomes might include.

- Improved teamworking in your practice.
- Better understanding of tasks required.
- Improved services for patients.

How would you demonstrate that you have achieved your outcomes?
An increased number of quality points in the identified areas for change.

Table 3.1: Role and responsibilities checklist – *for each task tick the box for each team member who has a role or responsibility – then note your role and responsibilities for the task*

Completed by: _____

Task	Primary care team member								What are your roles and your responsibilities?
	Doctor	Practice nurse	Receptionist team	HCAs	Practice manager	Practice secretary	Patient	Other	
Identifying areas for study and change	✔	✔	✔	✔	✔		✔		*e.g. Providing improved access for patients to health professionals*
Task 2									
Task 3									
Task 4									
Task 5									

Example problem case 2

Problem Case:

At a practice meeting, the practice secretary complains that there are large numbers of paper medical records in her office belonging to patients new to the practice. She says that she does not have time to put them in order, before they are passed on to the doctors, and the doctors will not tackle them until this is done. Her role is to transfer items highlighted by the doctors as important to go on the computerised record but she is struggling to do this because of other demands on her time. She says that other arrangements must be made.

Who do you need in your team?

You might want a team that includes:

Reception staff
Practice manager
Clerical and secretarial staff
Practice nurses
Healthcare assistants (HCAs)
Doctors
Patients.

Where you are now

This situation is seriously delaying access to the medical records of new patients, with its potential risks of lack of access to their previous medical history and treatment. The doctors say that they have enough to do and find it difficult to find time just to go through the records with a highlighting pen. Also, the secretary is much quicker at typing and finding the right Read codes.

What you do next

This might include the following.

- The practice manager asking for volunteers to put the records in date order.
- The practice manager identifying senior receptionists for training in Read coding entries.
- People at the meeting cannot identify any spare time for receptionists to do extra tasks, so the practice manager agrees to ask a retired member of staff who does holiday relief to do some extra hours in reception while training takes place.
- A course on Read coding is identified by the practice manager and staff are given paid time to attend. One of the doctors also agrees to go to become an expert resource for the other doctors. He becomes known as the 'Read police' by his partners as he corrects their coding entries!

- It is agreed that the identified senior receptionists will have practical training in rotation on coding entries. The practice manager and the secretary will be available for supervision and queries.
- One of the healthcare assistants says she would like to extend her skills by learning coding. She would like to increase her hours of work from just mornings back to full days. As she was previously one of the reception staff, she is included in the learning group and her hours of work and duties are re-negotiated.
- The doctors agree to take equal batches of new patient records once they have been organised into date order, to highlight important diagnoses, problems, treatments and allergies for entry on the computer.

What extra resources might this require?

- Temporary extra cover for reception staff learning to code.
- Cover for the receptionists attending the Read coding course.
- Re-grading of salaries to reflect the improved skills of senior reception staff.
- Designated time for the practice manager and secretary to help the receptionists to learn coding.
- More time on reception duties covered longer-term by the extra hours worked by the HCA.
- Time for the doctors to read through the paper records and summarise the medical history, where this has not been done by a previous practice.

The outcomes

The outcomes might include.

- Computerised records of significant past diagnosis, problems, treatment and allergies are available more quickly after patient registration, reducing risk.
- Senior receptionists feel that their skills are being recognised and extended and that they are making a more expert contribution to the practice.
- The secretary can concentrate on keeping coding entries up to date and on her other duties once training is completed.
- The doctors become more confident and accurate in their coding skills.

How would you demonstrate that you have achieved your outcomes?

- An audit shows that almost all paper medical records received by the practice are computerised within a reasonable time, e.g. four weeks.
- A review of coding entries by the 'expert' GP shows more accurate coding of diagnoses by the doctors.

Problem case exercise

> **Problem Case:**
>
> Last year at a meeting of all the practice team to look at future plans, the
> practice nurse said she would like to go on a course about spirometry
> organised by a pharmaceutical company. The senior partner was dismissive
> of her plans. He said that the practice did not need spirometry, it was going
> to be done by the hospital clinic and he didn't want pharmaceutical
> company interference in his prescribing. The practice nurse was upset and
> felt that her efforts to improve her skills were being blocked.
>
> This year the practice manager wants to avoid such confrontation. She wants
> to try and identify what the practice needs in the way of development and what
> services staff could develop. She makes plans to establish this before the meeting.

Who do you need in your team?

Where you are now

What you do next

Continued

What extra resources might this require?

The outcomes

How would you demonstrate that you have achieved your outcomes?

Identifying your learning needs

Personal responsibility

Each person is responsible for completing their own learning needs assessment, their own learning and making changes that are agreed as a practice organisation.

Responsibility as a practice organisation

Look at practice profiles, health needs assessments, clinical audits, staff appraisals and other forms of practice data to make sure these are up to date. Use several methods to identify your learning needs and/or gaps in your service development or delivery, so that you validate the findings of one method by another. No one method will give you reliable information about the gaps in your knowledge, skills or attitudes or everyday service.[1] Agree with members of your practice team your overall practice goals for chronic disease management and the role that each person can play.

Thinking about structural change

Make the structural changes required so that staff can put their learning into practice. For example, if someone is taking on new roles and responsibilities is this reflected in their job description? Separate out individuals' learning needs from other structural or resource needs that your practice may have, in order to effect change and improvements to patient care.[2]

In-house sessions

Organise two separate learning sessions in your practice to identify and prioritise what you need to learn about and what improvements you need to make to the services you provide. Include a representative from every team or group of staff within the practice organisation. Learning needs assessment helps you to match what you think you *want* to know as an individual and what you and others *need* to know.[2]

In the preliminary session you might:

- discuss how to assess individuals' learning needs
- decide how to collect data about your organisational readiness as a practice
- think how you will rank individual practice members' learning needs in order of priority
- consider people's personal learning styles and the type of learning activities needed
- develop a plan for analysing your learning needs in relation to chronic disease management over say, a four-week period.

In the second in-house session you might:

- enable individuals to discuss the data collected about people's learning needs and draft their learning plans
- help the practice team (or sub-teams) identify opportunities and potential barriers
- make an action plan and prioritise learning – all in relation to chronic disease management.

Assessment of learning needs in the practice team

Use a variety of methods over the course of time, to ensure on-going interest, and to try and avoid missing 'blind spots'. Look at Table 3.2 to help you formulate the questions you might want to ask.

Table 3.2:   Practice learning needs assessment (adapted from Bee and Bee[2])

Stage	Questions to ask in a team discussion	Process
1 Identifying the needs of the organisation	What are they?	Environmental scan: *External factors*: e.g. patients'/clients' unmet needs, current health policies, changing working practices, identified best practice, etc. *Internal factors*: e.g. staff – current and anticipated roles, responsibilities, areas of interest, readiness for and commitment to change.
2 Identifying and specifying learning needs	What are your performance needs? Where are your performance gaps? What changes are required to meet your performance needs? *Which* of these performance changes will be best met by the selected learning programmes?	Establishing current performance, identifying the gaps and establishing where learning can help. Consider using: • practice profiles/data/management information systems • performance management/appraisal • analysis of role specifications • succession planning • significant event analysis.
3 Planning the learning	Choose which chronic disease management areas are high priority. Which learning activities will be appropriate for which member(s)/staff group(s) within your practice organisation? What is your practice-based learning plan for using this programme?	Include in the learning plan: • staff requiring different aspects of learning programme • plans for sharing learning amongst team and wider • main aims and objectives for learning • planned timescale • methods for evaluating the learning against your organisational needs.
4 Evaluating the learning	Has the learning been effective in helping you to meet your identified goals and outcomes?	1 *Short term:* • initial thoughts and feelings • satisfaction with the learning programme • knowledge and skills acquired during programme. 2 *Intermediate:* • how has learning affected the way team members perform in their roles? 3 *Long term:* • how has learning helped practice organisation meet its needs in managing chronic disease?

Identifying external factors

An environmental scan

You can carry out a political, economic, sociological and technical (PEST) analysis (*see* Box 3.1).[3] Discuss and list the political, economic, sociological and technological factors that influence your practice's aims and objectives in respect of chronic disease management. It can also help to isolate those factors for which the practice organisation carries direct responsibility from those that are outside of its direct control.

Box 3.1:   PEST analysis[3]

Political: Economic:

Sociological: Technological:

Identifying internal factors

Analysing your strengths, weaknesses, opportunities and threats (SWOT) will help to illuminate organisational strengths and weaknesses in relation to current chronic disease management in your practice.[3] It should help you to identify any gaps between your aims for effective chronic disease management by your practice team, and your current performance. Share these ideas within the whole team. Consider data from the following sources.

- **Practice profiles and health needs assessment**: e.g. demography of patient population, epidemiology (ask your local public health department to supply information), high-risk groups of patients, hospital admission rates, current provision of care or services.
- **Clinical audits**: are current indicators and benchmarks in chronic disease management being met such as those in the quality and outcomes framework?
- **Performance management/staff appraisal**: to determine your team's strengths, weaknesses and personal development needs.
- **Patient/user surveys**: that you have carried out, or the PCO or NHS has done on your patients.
- **Analysis of the current roles of the team**: compare current team roles with where you are aiming to be with effective chronic disease management. Have you thought about succession planning for your expert practice nurses for instance?

- **Significant event analysis**: what issues and needs are emerging from these?
- **Practice complaints**.
- **Patients and/or carers**: invite them to an educational or planning session with your team.
- **NHS policy and guidelines**: consider how they relate to the way you are running your practice.

Involve everyone in developing your aims

Patient and public involvement in planning and delivering healthcare is a central component of healthcare policy. The closer you are to consulting users of your services, the better able you will be to identify their needs and preferences and go on to provide more appropriate services.[4] Try to ensure that the input of individual patients is representative of the relevant patient groups.[5]

Identifying performance gaps

After undertaking some of these exercises, start identifying gaps between your practice team's current performance in chronic disease management, and where it needs to be to meet your aims. Consider what you can alter by arranging learning activities for team members and what may need a reallocation of resources, or organisational, structural or cultural changes. Learning cannot be effective without taking account of all of these.[2] Try completing Box 3.2 for each of your identified aims.

Box 3.2: Integrating learning – overall practice organisational aims for the delivery of effective chronic disease management				
Objectives (in order of priority)	Learning required	Resources required/ reallocated	Organisational/ structural changes required	Cultural change required

Self-assess your learning needs as an individual

Looking at your role and responsibilities within the practice organisation helps you to assess your learning needs. You can identify areas of strengths and weaknesses in your knowledge, skills and attitudes and develop a personal learning plan. This should contribute to the overall practice learning plan, in this case in relation to chronic disease management. You can use the activities described above, and others, for individual assessment of need.[6-8]

Knowing your personal learning style is an important element of preparing yourself for learning. Honey and Mumford's learner style inventory is often used to help classify someone's personal learning style.[9] Then you can match the way you learn (attend a course or small group, read, observe, practice, etc.) with what suits your own style.

You might use several methods to establish your own learning needs such as:

- constructive feedback from colleagues or patients (planned or informal)
- chats and discussion with members of your practice team
- 360 degree feedback
- self-assessment, or review by others, using a rating scale to assess your skills and attitudes
- comparison with protocols and guidelines for checking how well procedures are followed
- audit: various types and applications
- significant event audit
- eliciting patient views such as satisfaction surveys
- a SWOT (strengths, weaknesses, opportunities and threats) analysis
- reading and reflecting
- problem case analysis
- educational review.[10,11]

Several of these methods will also be useful for identifying team development needs – you can look at the gaps identified from both the personal and team perspectives at the same time using the same method, e.g. SWOT analysis.

Thinking about evaluation

Evaluate whether learning has made a difference to the performance gaps you initially identified from individual and organisational perspectives. Different levels of evaluation are presented in Box 3.3.

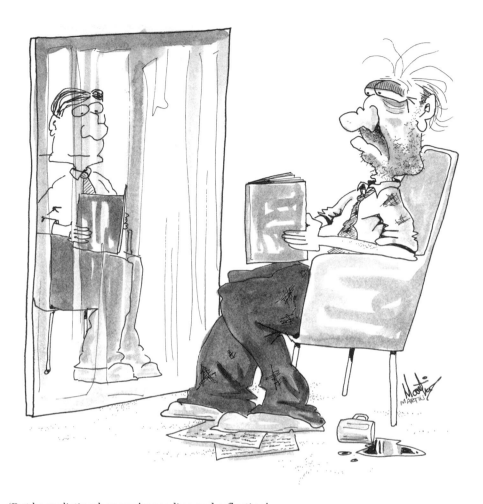

'But be realistic when you're reading and reflecting'

Box 3.3:   Levels of evaluation[2,3]

Evaluation level	**Questions to ask from individual and organisational perspectives**
1 Evaluation of reaction: immediate, on completion of the learning programme	What I/we liked and why What I/we disliked and why What I/we have learnt What areas am I/are we still uncertain about and how can we improve this?
2 Learning and performance levels of evaluation (at approximately three months following completion of programme)	Have I/we achieved our objectives for learning in knowledge, skill and behaviour? How is the learning transferring into practice? How can we assess whether this has been achieved? This could be achieved for example, through using practice observation, peer review or reflective practice as well as through performance appraisal.
3 Evaluation of results completed several months after the learning has taken place	What were our original aims? What was the baseline data that contributed to our needs analysis? What indicators will demonstrate a change in performance and identify whether our aims have been achieved? Examples might include: • reduction in patients with chronic diseases being admitted to hospital • increase in nurse-led services • reduction in patient complaints • more frequent multidisciplinary team meetings.

Readiness of the organisation for providing a learning climate

The work environment in your practice is an important influence in terms of facilitating or inhibiting learning.[6] Some key factors that can promote your practice workplace as an effective learning environment follow.

Symbiotic leadership

Four key activities that leaders and managers need to undertake to develop a supportive learning climate within their organisation are:

1 role modelling
2 providing opportunities to learn
3 building learning into the organisational processes
4 acting as learning champions.[6]

Use the checklist in Box 3.4 to look at whether leaders in your practice actively facilitate learning for others.

Box 3.4: Leaders and the learning climate		
In my practice/team do I: Provide opportunities for staff to observe and reflect upon good role modelling, e.g. shadowing, peer observation, reflective discourse?	**Yes**	**No**
Select and provide learning opportunities for myself and for others in my team or practice?		
Provide opportunities for learning in our team activities, e.g. do we meet regularly and allow time for discussion and reflection after team meetings?		
Treat learning as a priority within our practice organisation and encourage and empower others to use teaching and learning opportunities?		

Project teams

Learning through focusing on specific projects can help to develop critical enquiry skills throughout your practice team. Working and reflecting in teams can also help individuals to be creative and innovative in their jobs and learn together within the workplace (*see* Chapter 2).

Culture and climate

Setting up a culture with an egalitarian philosophy means that everyone is valued for his or her contribution to, and views about, the practice organisation. Developing reflective behaviour within your practice is an important step in this process.[11] Providing opportunities to learn new roles and responsibilities and develop career paths can provide a challenging work environment and stimulate learning for team members. Organisational leaders, such as the practice manager or GP(s), should constantly monitor and review the aims, priorities and outcomes in relation to effective chronic disease management, in the light of the rapidly changing healthcare context.

Learning and service outcomes

What are the pitfalls?

You need to consider the blocks and barriers to learning that may be present in your practice organisation. These may include poor communication, tribalism, and dominance of some team members over others, lack of shared ownership and lack of needs assessment before learning.[3]

Look at the questions in Box 3.5. You might ask each member of the practice team to complete this questionnaire so that you get a comprehensive review. Alternatively, sub-teams within the practice organisation could use this tool to guide a group discussion on your learning climate.

Box 3.5: Considering the learning climate	Yes	No
Do all members of your team feel valued for their contribution to the practice team/organisation – even those who work on the periphery?		
Is there good communication within your team even with members who work in relative isolation or who work part-time?		
Do different disciplines within the team value changing roles and responsibilities?		
Do team members take personal responsibility for their self-directed learning or are they reluctant to use 'learner centred', interactive approaches to learning?		
Are all team members allowed dedicated time for learning?		
Is there a system for appraising personal learning needs so that learning can be appropriately targeted?		

Look at what needs to change in order to overcome any particular barrier to learning within your practice organisation and identify an appropriate action plan for change as in Box 3.6.

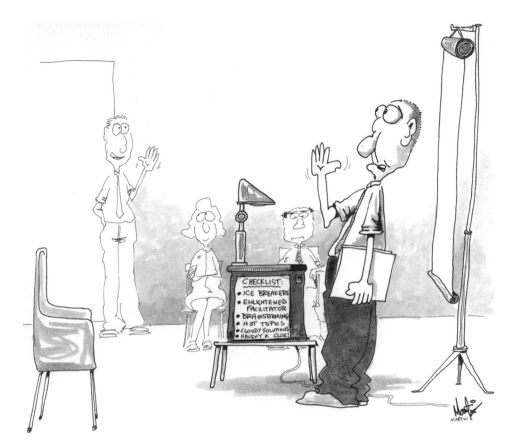

Learning climate

What you can do to make it likely you will succeed

The following activities will help both individuals and the practice as a whole learn about effective chronic disease management.[12,13] Think whether this is current practice or if changes should be made to provide an optimum learning environment in your workplace.

- Encourage learning equally for all.
- Think about how those learning new knowledge, skills and attitudes can have the chance to practise new behaviours within a safe environment. Mentorship and clinical supervision should help to improve the support to individuals.
- Do not give colleagues or yourself too much to learn at one time – be aware that different team members will learn at different speeds.
- Try to ensure that the learning that is being expected of individuals is relevant and meaningful for them and that everyone in the practice understands the importance of this learning.
- Think how the capabilities and skills of staff can be fully enhanced – not only through learning but also in their role structure and responsibilities.
- Provide regular opportunities for staff to learn together in teams, particularly in a problem-based or project-focused way.

Box 3.6: Organisational learning plan

Organisational aim	Organisational objective	Appropriate chronic disease management unit	Appropriate for	To be completed by

- Establish a non-threatening environment in which individual members of your team can allow their assumptions to be challenged.
- Work together as a practice team or organisation to develop and share a cohesive vision.
- Think about how the work you are doing as a practice organisation fits into the wider organisational picture and the whole system of care as experienced by the patients using your practice.

Having identified your learning needs as a practice team, look at which elements of the chronic disease management programme could help you to meet those needs. You might use Box 3.6 to categorise your aims, the staff involved and the date by which learning should be completed.

References

1 Chambers R, Wakley G and variety of other authors (2004) *Demonstrating Your Competence. Series of Books 1–5* (for GPs and nurses). Radcliffe Publishing, Oxford.

2 Bee F and Bee R (2003) *Learning Needs Analysis and Evaluation.* Chartered Institute of Personnel Development, London.

3 Garcarz W, Chambers R and Ellis S (2003) *Make Your Healthcare Organisation a Learning Organisation.* Radcliffe Medical Press, Oxford.

4 Crowley P, Green J, Freake D *et al.* (2002) Primary Care Trusts involving the community: is community development the way forward? *Journal of Management in Medicine.* **16(4)**: 311–22.

5 Chambers R, Drinkwater C and Boath E (2003) *Involving Patients and the Public: how to do it better* (2e). Radcliffe Medical Press, Oxford.

6 Lideway EC (2004) Designing the workplace for learning and innovation. *Development and Learning in Organisations.* **18(5)**: 10–13.

7 Grant J (2002) Learning needs assessment: assessing the need. *BMJ.* **324**: 156–9.

8 Wakley G, Chambers R and Field S (2000) *Continuing Professional Development in Primary Care: making it happen.* Radcliffe Medical Press, Oxford.

9 Honey P and Mumford A (1992) *The Manual of Learning Styles.* Peter Honey, Maidenhead.

10 Chambers R (ed.) (2002) *A Guide to Accredited Professional Development.* Royal College of General Practitioners, London.

11 Chambers R and Wakley G (2005) *Clinical Audit in Primary Care: demonstrating quality and outcomes.* Radcliffe Publishing, Oxford.

12 Rushmer R, Kelly D, Lough M *et al.* (2004) Introducing the Learning Practice – 1. The characteristics of learning organisations in primary care. *Evaluation in Clinical Practice.* **10(2)**: 375–86.

13 Rushmer R, Kelly D, Lough M *et al.* (2004) Introducing the Learning Practice – II. Becoming a learning practice. *Evaluation in Clinical Practice.* **10(3)**: 387–98.

4

Organising chronic disease management to match the quality and outcomes framework

The quality and outcomes framework (QOF) for general practice is voluntary and general practice teams can decide whether to enter and which levels they wish to achieve.[1] Payments are linked to achievement of the individual criteria and standards. Each criterion has a number of points allocated to it. The number of points varies according to the amount and difficulty of the work required to achieve success with each criterion.

The whole document is called a framework. It is organised into four domains: clinical, organisational, patient experience and additional services (*see* Table 4.1). Each domain is divided into a number of areas. Each area is subdivided into individual indicators, the audit criteria.

The points from the four domains add up to 1000 points. A further 50 points are available for the access payment. A monetary amount is attached to each area for a payment to the practice. The financial amount is based on the average practice of 5500 patients and three GP principals. The payment to practices is proportionately adjusted for the notional number of patients to be treated. This is done using a formula. The formula will be adjusted as information about disease prevalence is improved. The notional number of patients to be treated is related to the difficulty and workload expected to produce high-quality care. Disease registers of the clinical domain will in time reveal the prevalence and influences on disease prevalence.

Table 4.1: Structure of the quality and outcomes framework[1]

	Domain			
	Clinical	*Organisational*	*Patient experience*	*Additional services*
Areas in each domain	Ten clinical areas	Five organisational areas	Two areas	Four clinical areas that practices can choose to be involved with to a specified standard

Clinical domain

The clinical domain is constructed using clinical criteria and standards in ten areas.

1   Coronary heart disease (CHD) including left ventricular dysfunction (LVD)
2   Stroke and transient ischaemic attack (TIA)
3   Hypertension
4   Hypothyroidism
5   Diabetes
6   Mental health
7   Chronic obstructive pulmonary disease (COPD)
8   Asthma
9   Epilepsy
10 Cancer.

The criteria are summative and the vast majority of the data can be collected from the computer system. This will produce a uniform measurement method, clarity, and accurate ranking between practices of outcomes without specifying what process has been used. Box 4.1 summarises the stages in the process of reaching the key components of the process.

Box 4.1:   Principles of the clinical domain

- Accurate and complete disease register
- Measure the criterion
- Upper and lower level standards for each criterion
- Measure control of the disease
- Variable maximum control levels for each criterion
- Exclusion of patients for patient choice and clinical reasons

---

Your practice is required to create an accurate register for the disease in question. The indicators for each clinical area are described. For each there is a standard. This represents the upper level for which payments are available. For the criteria that specify process measures, for example the measurement of blood pressure, there is a common standard of 90% achievement. For the outcome measures, for example control of blood pressure to below 150/90, individual standards have been set. If the patient refuses to have treatment, they can be excluded from the population for that particular criterion. Practices can only *request* patients to make changes to the way they look after themselves or co-operate with treatment. Patients should be informed about the options and be able to make a choice. For individual criteria there may be other specific exclusions mentioned in the guidance or agreed at the time of the assessment visit by the PCO. It is believed that standards can be reached without describing exclusions for all criteria. So, if the practice has achieved the levels there is no need to discuss exclusions but the option remains if there are good reasons for not reaching the standard.

Organisational domain

The organisational criteria are designed to achieve two functions. Firstly, they list tasks that are required to prove compliance with legislation or good practice. Secondly, they signpost the organisational tasks required to improve best practice. Box 4.2 lists the key principles upon which the organisational domain is based.

Box 4.2:   Principles of the organisational framework

- Criteria are developmental so that they can be achieved gradually
- All practices should reach a minimum standard
- Measurable in a simple and reliable way
- Points (and resources) allocated in proportion to the difficulty of the task
- Some criteria function as markers to show that generic skills are present in the practice
- The generic skills should be used to improve the way that the practice carries out other work
- Success with the criteria achieves clinical governance requirements

---

The criteria are divided into five areas. Each criterion is separately scored for points. This allows practices to develop at different speeds with different domains yet reduce the complexity of the payment system. The five domains are.

1   Records and information about patients
2   Communicating with patients
3   Education and training
4   Practice management
5   Medicines management.

Patient experience domain

The domain for 'patient experience' is intended to allow the practice to look at how patients view the practice. The practice can ask patients for their opinions and meet patient needs. A choice of tools has been agreed and others could be added later. Box 4.3 describes the principles underpinning this domain.

Box 4.3:   Principles required in the patient experience

- Consultation with patients by questionnaire
- Acting on results
- Practices not ranked by the values obtained
- Aim is to inform practices of their own patients' requests

Patient questionnaires

Two patient questionnaires, the General Practice Assessment Questionnaire (GPAQ) and the Improving Practices Questionnaire (IPQ) have been accepted as valid measures of patient views. Issue these to patients on an annual basis. You can post the questionnaires or give them out to patients in the surgery. They aim to look at the experience of the practice that is not measured by the clinical and organisational standards. The questionnaires look specifically at access, the quality of the consultation itself and the information given out, the quality of the premises and other parts of the practice that patients have experienced.

The questionnaires are standardised and have been used extensively in British general practice. The GPAQ instrument is free to use and printed copies can be obtained for a fee. The IPQ instrument is not free but the cost includes printed questionnaires and analysis.

The General Medical Services (GMS) contract requires the practice to:

• use a patient questionnaire
• prepare a report, draw inferences from the results and take action
• discuss the anonymised results with a third party representing either patients or the primary care organisation.

In this way, the views of patients are fed back to the practice and increasing use made of their input. Practices are not scored according to the absolute values of the results and patients' views do not affect income.

Appointment length

The contract rewards the use of ten-minute appointment length for routine consultations and you should be able to demonstrate that this time is usually available.

Consulting with patients about other issues

The contract does not require you to ask patients about other experiences but as practices become used to the concept of consulting patients, refinements may be introduced in addition to, or in place of, the two named questionnaires.

Additional medical services

Not all practices will provide additional medical services. The areas covered are.

1   Cervical screening
2   Child health surveillance
3   Maternity services
4   Contraceptive services.

Most of the criteria in these areas require the creation of, or adherence to, local policies. Only cervical cytology is summative and has a standard. All are areas that attracted separate payments under the old GMS contract. There is no gradation for partial achievement except cervical cytology, and points are awarded for agreeing to provide the service. If practices choose not to provide these services, the PCO can provide or purchase them elsewhere based on the same criteria.

Contractual and statutory requirements

The GMS contract contains twenty-five additional organisational criteria, quite separate from the QOF. These specify minimum standards for the practice. They are not voluntary and no payments attach to them. They apply irrespective of whether the practice decides to participate in the QOF.

They are a mix of restatements of the law and established working practices in the NHS. All should be happening now but it is worth reviewing the criteria themselves to check that you are working to them. Some require the creation of policies. Many are worded to suggest adherence to legislation and practices that will change with time. There are no standards because complete achievement is required. Where information is required, it should be readily available from the named statutory organisation or the PCO.

Using information technology to help achieve quality

Information technology (IT) is a tool to help achieve quality and quality criteria. It is about the people who operate the systems and what they have to be able to do to help the practice achieve quality.

Practice responsibilities

The cost of staff to operate the systems is a practice responsibility and paid for out of practice resources. The ability to use the practice computer system in-house will profoundly affect performance on the clinical indicators of the QOF.

It is extremely difficult to achieve high levels in the clinical domain without extensive use of a computerised database in the practice. Whilst there is no necessity for practices to enter data in specific ways, it is much easier to enter data accurately and in the right place using a template and the same Read code for the same illness. It is likely that computer systems will produce prompts and practices will produce protocols for how they would like data to be entered. It will be a practice decision how to clean the database and which staff members are most appropriate to do that.

The contractual and statutory requirements specify that the practice has to maintain good computer use in accordance with current legislation. This requires the practice to have someone responsible for confidentiality, and confidentiality has to be explained to patients. The practice must be registered for data protection and make electronic data available to the next practice for patients moving between practices. Practice staff need to be able to perform the tasks in Box 4.4 and the database needs to be accurate.

Box 4.4:   Practice IT tasks

- Cleaning the database
- Entering data recorded in paper records on to the computer
- Training professionals in data entry
- Learning to add data at the time of the consultation
- Entering data for many illnesses at one consultation
- Training staff in audit
- Carrying out audits at intervals during the year to establish how well the practice is doing
- Call and recall of patients with missing data or partially controlled diseases
- Preparing data for submission at the end of the year

Cleaning and improving existing data

In many practices in the past, data has been collected as *written* records and not entered on computers. If the practice has been controlling blood pressures and treating hypertension well but not recording it, the task is to improve the recording of data, not to change treatment. Experience elsewhere has shown that improving the recording of missing data by searching notes for data can result in rapid improvements in computerised records. Computer staff can enter this data, as it does not require input from clinicians.

To target this work compile a disease index on the computer then search that group of patients on the disease register to see if the parameter, say blood pressure, has been recorded in the past year. This can then be added to the computerised register if present on the paper record. It is more economical in time and effort to look for several parameters, e.g. blood pressure, smoking habits, smoking cessation, results of measurements such as blood glucose or cholesterol, etc., and update the electronic records for diabetes, CHD and other diseases at one time. Templates help to structure the collection of data. Computer records for results from blood tests are automatically recorded if they are gathered over an electronic link. In time, other clinical parameters like blood pressure taken in secondary care will be added to the practice record directly too.

Existing disease indexes are not always accurate. Sometimes inaccurate diagnoses have been recorded in the past. Each entry needs to be checked either from the records or in a consultation. Patients will usually know if they have had an illness. Do this 'cleaning' of disease registers early on. Some patients with illnesses may not have a diagnosis recorded. It may be impossible to rectify this easily other than by summarising the medical records and transferring the patient information in Read coded form to the computer. Repeat medication provides a ready way of identifying patients on medication for many illnesses such as CHD or depression.

Improving quality of new data entry

Improving the quality of data entry requires clinicians to enter data at every relevant consultation for each parameter. It is often easier to enter the data into a template on the computer than to try to remember what to add. This also encourages use of common Read codes in standard situations. The template should record the important data and not record other data of less importance that is not required for every patient. Entering past morbidity data during consultations takes up considerable time but rapidly improves disease indexes.

Auditing the current situation

Once the database has been cleaned and the disease indexes reflect the number of patients with particular illnesses, the practice can start to improve the quality of clinical care. For some practices the quality of chronic disease management is already good and only fine-tuning will be required. Effort can then be focused elsewhere. For others action on clinical management will be required.

Use your computer records to find out which patients should be recalled for the review (usually annual) required by many of the criteria in the QOF. These reviews can be run in conjunction with the repeat prescription system. As medication reviews are completed, relevant information about other aspects of the patient's care can be collected and added to the computer record.

Use your computer for specific searches, then print off letters to patients to request that they attend the surgery or supply the information required to complete their records. For this you need sufficient trained staff, an accurate database and adequate terminals for someone to be able to search the database. This type of search can be run either in the clinical system or in a separate software system.

Plan improvements to the way your practice is organised

Use the matrix in Table 4.2 to record a baseline in your practice, for who is able to do what in respect of the clinical domain, or how individual team member's responsibilities are being carried out. Where your audit shows gaps in the way you are doing things in your practice, make plans for improvement. Now move on to audit the quality and completeness of records and information about patients in Table 4.3. Complete the action points for who will be responsible for changes that need to be made in the tables.

Draw-up your educational plan and revisit your business plan for the practice

When you have completed Table 4.4 reflect and discuss as a practice team what you need to do to underpin your service improvements with learning activities and evolve an educational plan for the team. Look back at Chapter 3 to read more about this. You could centre your plan on PBL sessions run in your practice using this series of chronic disease management learning.

Table 4.2: Planning to achieve clinical criteria

Organisational requirement	Is it happening already?	Who should do the task?	Responsible person?	Structural change required?	Skills required?	Training or course required?
Clinical criteria						
IT						
Cleaning the disease registers						
Adding to the disease registers						
Entering data to the computer already recorded in the paper records						
Seeing the patients requiring care						
Number and nature of disease management clinics						
Writing practice policies						
Writing patient group directions						
Number of additional doctors required						
Number of additional nurses required						
Number of additional team members, e.g. pharmacist						
Infrastructure implications						
Number of computer terminals						
Capacity of central server, IT system provider						
Nature of computer peripherals, back-up method, printers, other software available						
Number of receptionists required						
Demand for prescriptions						
Management support for the larger practice						
Staff (changes are present in organisational criteria)						

Table 4.3: Planning to achieve organisational criteria

Records and information about patients	Is it happening already?	Who should do the task?	Responsible person?	Structural change required?	Skills required?	Training or course required?
Organisational standard						
Each patient contact with a clinician is recorded in the patient's record, including consultations, visits and telephone advice						
Entries in the records are legible						
The practice has a system for transferring and acting on information about patients seen by other doctors out of hours						
There is a reliable system to ensure that messages and requests for visits are recorded and that the appropriate doctor or team member receives and acts upon them						
The practice has a system for dealing with any hospital report or investigation results which identifies a responsible health professional and ensures that any necessary action is taken						
There is a system for ensuring that the relevant team members are informed about patients who have died						
The medicines that a patient is receiving are clearly listed in their record						
There is a designated place for the recording of drug allergies and adverse reactions in the notes and these are clearly recorded						
For repeat medication, an indication for the drug can be identified in the records (for drugs added to repeat prescription with effect from 1 April 2004)						

Continued

Table 4.3: *continued*

Records and information about patients	Is it happening already?	Who should do the task?	Responsible person?	Structural change required?	Skills required?	Training or course required?
The smoking status of patients aged 15–75 years is recorded						
The blood pressure of patients aged 45 years and over is recorded in preceding five years						
When a member of the team prescribes a medication other than a non-medicated dressing, topical treatment, or over-the-counter medication, there is a mechanism for that prescription to be entered into the patient's general practice record						
There is a system to alert the out-of-hours service or duty doctor to patients dying at home						
The records, hospital letters and investigation reports are filed in date order, or available electronically in date order						
The practice has up-to-date clinical summaries						
Newly registered patients have had their notes summarised within eight weeks of receipt by the practice						

Table 4.4: Planning to achieve criteria common to several domains through learning and investment

Organisational requirement	Is it happening already?	Who should do the task?	Responsible person?	Structural change required?	Skills required?	Training or course required?
Common requirements across all domains						
Education requirement						
Creating a practice professional development plan						
Requirement for education meetings						
Business planning						
Creating a business plan						
Requirement for planning meetings						

Include the resource implications of service improvements when you are working through the problems in your practice for the various chronic diseases. You need to revise or create your practice business plan to invest in improving your services, in response to the audits you have logged in Tables 4.2 and 4.3 and other gaps you identify in meeting your quality and outcomes framework indicators.

Clinical audit

Clinical audit is the method used by health professionals to assess, improve and evaluate the care of patients in a systematic way, to enhance their health and quality of life. It is key to demonstrating the extent to which a practice has attained the criteria compared to the standards as set out in the quality and outcomes framework, which are then translated into points, and points translated into practice income. The steps of any audit cycle are to:

1 describe the domain, criteria and standards you are trying to achieve
2 measure your current performance of how well you are providing care or services in an objective way
3 compare your performance against criteria and standards – as described in the QOF
4 identify the need for change – to performance, of criteria or standards, resources, available data
5 make any required changes as necessary – as in the three righthand columns in Tables 4.2, 4.3 and 4.4
6 re-audit later.

Example: developing a practice-based system for providing effective care for left ventricular dysfunction

The GMS contract has criteria for left ventricular dysfunction (LVD) but there is also other guidance and a wider set of requirements to treat the disease available from other national sources such as the National Institute for Clinical Excellence (NICE) and Scottish Intercollegiate Guidelines Network (SIGN).

Defining the illness

Look at NICE guidelines[2] or the similar SIGN website[3] to define the domain. There is also authoritative guidance in the publication *Clinical Evidence*.[4] Increasingly, evidence is collated at the National electronic Library for Health.[5]

Prepare a short report on LVD for your practice so you all know what you are dealing with, and have a practice policy that matches with the local hospital policy, and complete Table 4.2. Describe the components of LVD as in Box 4.5. This should be presented in a written and/or electronic format(s). Laminated pages may be pinned on consulting room walls and/or as templates on the practice computer (*see* Chapter 10 for more information about LVD).

Box 4.5: Components of the definition of a chronic disease

Describe:

- diagnostic names used
- clinical syndromes themselves
- tests required to make the diagnosis
- different grades of the disease
- standard treatment (for different grades of the illness)
- regular monitoring required (for different grades of the illness)
- relevant Read codes

Improving the service for LVD in the practice

Assuming that you have worked as a practice to create and clean up disease registers, improved your use of IT to search for patients and call them up for regular reviews, you will now focus on the care you are providing for patients with LVD. The requirements of the GMS contract for LVD are listed in Table 4.5.

Table 4.5: Quality and outcome measures for left ventricular dysfunction

Domain		Percentage threshold (minimum 25%) (%)	Points
LVD 1:	The practice can produce a register of patients with CHD and left ventricular dysfunction		4
LVD 2:	The percentage of patients with a diagnosis of CHD and left ventricular dysfunction (diagnosed after 1/4/03) which has been confirmed by echocardiogram	90	6
LVD 3:	The percentage of patients with a diagnosis of CHD and left ventricular dysfunction who are currently treated with ACE inhibitors (or A2 antagonists)	70	10

As in Table 4.2, decide which tasks a doctor needs to do and which tasks others should or could do. Decide who is to do what as well as what is to be done.

In order to confirm LVD, a 12-lead ECG and/or a brain natriuretic peptide test should be abnormal. If either is abnormal, an echocardiogram should then be arranged. The GP contract requires an echocardiogram to confirm the diagnosis of left ventricular systolic dysfunction for patients suspected of having LVD after 1/4/03. Some computer software mistakenly puts a new date in if the diagnosis is re-entered. Dates of diagnosis must be accurate.

Once the diagnosis is confirmed, treatment is required. NICE guidance suggests diuretics, angiotensin-converting enzyme (ACE) inhibitors, certain beta blockers, spironolactone (for a sub-group) and digoxin. The contract requires audit data for the use of ACE inhibitors and angiotensin-II (A2) receptor antagonists (Box 4.6). The practice team can decide if it wishes to audit its achievement of other parameters too.

If all patients have been started and remain on the correct treatment, the monitoring software or audits will show complete achievement of the criteria. This is unlikely!

Box 4.6:   Initial audits

1   Collate number of patients with LVD (note the Read code is for left ventricular failure – LVF – as no code for LVD exists)
2   Decide if this is an accurate reflection of expected numbers of LVD. Will searching for ACE inhibitors or diuretics produce more patients with the diagnosis?
3   Calculate the proportion of patients coded for LVD who were diagnosed after 1/4/03. Are the dates accurate?
4   Count how many patients diagnosed after 1/4/03 have had an echocardiogram or have been referred for an echocardiogram
5   Carry out an audit of what proportion of all patients with LVD are on ACE inhibitors or angiotensin-II receptor antagonists

---

Each of these audits will produce lists of named patients with tests or treatments that are not completed. A call and recall system for patients will be required to correct any deficiencies. The initial search will produce the number of patients requiring ECGs, echocardiograms and to be started on ACE inhibitors. If these tests are missing, the practice should send an invitation to consult a doctor or nurse in clinic to arrange the tests, if the administrative staff cannot arrange them, working to a protocol.

Once patients have been started on treatment, they will need regular review. This is not specified in the GMS contract but NICE guidance requires:

- assessment of functional capacity
- assessment of fluid status
- assessment of cardiac rhythm
- laboratory assessment (blood test monitoring).

This is in addition to the requirements to monitor ischaemic heart disease.

Making it happen

One of the clinicians in the practice team will probably take a lead on LVD. They will have learned about LVD and gradually have realised how much work is required. They will work out how much staff time is needed to make changes to practice systems as in Box 4.7. Then members of the practice team will have to change their working practices to deliver best practice care in relation to patients with LVD.

Box 4.7:   Producing a plan to improve the service for a chronic disease

Consider:

- What is the division of tasks between doctors, nurses and administrative staff?
- Which other areas of practice work will be affected by the change? For example, if a practice nurse runs a new clinic for this group, who will do the work she/he previously did?
- Are costs of new members of staff in the budget?
- Who is responsible for producing job specifications and appointing new members of staff?
- Who is responsible for training existing or new staff?

GPs and nurses in the practice have a significant impact on the way diagnoses are made and the clinical treatments that patients are given. The clinical lead for LVD will need to involve and inform the other clinicians as the practice protocol is drawn up to encourage their ownership. Then he or she will have to maintain colleagues' interest and commitment as well as encouraging them to stick with the changes agreed. This may require a concerted effort to sort out how the GPs and nurses work together as a really well functioning team, so that everyone agrees to adopt a consistent approach to managing each chronic disease, not just LVD as in this case.

The clinical lead should organise an educational event to challenge the team's existing views of treatment and present the reasons to change. Implementing NICE and other guidelines successfully requires an understanding and explanation of the issues in each individual practice and a desire to implement them.

References

1   General Practitioners Committee/The NHS Confederation (2003) *New GMS Contract. Investing in General Practice*. British Medical Association, London.

2   www.nice.org.uk

3   www.sign.ac.uk

4   Godlee F (ed.) (2004) *Clinical Evidence. Issue 11*. BMJ Publishing Group, London. www.clinicalevidence.com

5   www.nelh.nhs.uk

5

Diabetes

Review a case (or cases) with which your team has been involved to explore how your primary care team might work together to improve the management of patients with diabetes. You may prefer to use the two example cases at the start of this chapter. Read through them quickly before working on the problem case exercise (*see* page 71), or just photocopy Table 1.1 on page 7 to develop your own problem case. Include in your team, people who will join in the problem-based learning discussion and be part of the solutions.

If you feel that you have insufficient knowledge to guide you in completing the problem-based learning, use the summary about diabetes in the second part of this chapter and follow up the references if you need to learn more.

Example problem case 1

Problem Case:

The practice lead on diabetes is concerned to hear that the number of patients with diabetes on the practice register is considerably below that expected for the age, social class and ethnic composition of the practice population.

Who do you need in your team?

You might want a team that includes:

Patients and carers
Practice nurses
GPs
Clerical staff
Practice manager
District nurses
Pharmacist
Podiatrist
Optometrist
Cleaners.

Where you are now

The register for diabetes has evolved following a search for all patients on oral hypoglycaemic agents and insulin. It has been added to over the last two years by opportunistically recording patients with diabetes who are seen at home or in the surgery, or from hospital discharge letters – when people remember.

What you do next

This might include.

- Running an information campaign for patients and carers about the reasons for having a register of people with diabetes. Invite people with diabetes to ask if they are included on the disease register.
- Recording consistently all patients discharged from hospital with any diagnosis of diabetes.
- Asking the district nurses and podiatrists for details of all patients who they see who have diabetes.
- Producing a written policy of how a diagnosis of diabetes is made and how you differentiate between type 1 and type 2 diabetes.
- Running a search for all patients who are prescribed blood glucose monitoring equipment i.e. blood glucose test strips and lancets and urine test strips.
- Keeping a list of children with diabetes and transferring their names to the adult diabetic register when they reach 17 years of age.
- Asking the local pharmacist if they are willing to offer opportunistic or fasting, near testing blood sugar measurements to increase the pick-up rate of diabetes. Liaise with pharmacist over blood glucose monitoring and ensure that strips and lancets prescribed are compatible with patients' machines.
- Running a patient information session or two, with expert patient and health promotion staff input.
- Offering fasting blood glucose testing to anyone with a relative with diabetes or who has a body mass index (BMI) over 30.
- Completing Table 5.1.

What extra resources might this require?

- Time and expertise to produce a poster and leaflet campaign in the waiting room of the practice. Training for reception staff so that they can answer queries about services available to people with diabetes, and what safeguards to confidentiality exist.
- Train one or two clerical staff to identify any diagnosis of diabetes on patients' discharge letters and record the patients on the diabetic register. This will take them away from other practice activities and additional staff time may be needed.
- The district nurses will need training and secure access to the computer system if they are to add patients to the diabetic register. This involves time, access to a spare terminal and someone to train them. The time they spend takes them away from other tasks that still have to be done, so additional nursing time may be required. This training would be useful for other tasks, so could be justified on other grounds, e.g. for entering details of other care, or finding out necessary clinical information about patients under their care. The clerical staff above will need to

enter the data supplied by other team members such as podiatrists, and from the district nurses if they do not wish, or have no need, to access the computer system for other tasks.

- Time and resources for the practice team to produce an agreed written policy of how the diagnosis of diabetes is made.
- Clerical staff need time and training to keep a list of children with diabetes and add their names to the diabetic register when they reach 17 years of age.
- The local pharmacy would have to justify the outlay in commercial terms, e.g. increased business, if they are to offer opportunistic or fasting blood sugar measurements.
- A patient information session or two, with health promotion input requires time from all staff involved (doctor, practice nurse, health promotion staff), access to suitable premises (not necessarily the practice – a community venue might be better) and resources (patient literature, posters, etc.) as well as willing and suit-ably well-informed patients.
- Offering fasting blood glucose testing to anyone with a relative with diabetes or who has a BMI over 30 requires costing of resources in consumables and staff time.

The outcomes

The outcomes might include.

- Increased numbers of people identified correctly as having diabetes.
- Greater awareness of diabetes by patients and staff.
- Justification of the number of people on the diabetes register.
- Ability to maintain the diabetic register correctly in the future.
- A register from which other actions for diabetes care can be managed.

How would you demonstrate that you have achieved your outcomes?

A diabetic register that included the number of patients with diabetes expected from the age, social class and ethnic mix of the practice population.

(Please *see* Chapter 1 if you and your practice team would like to consider an example about type 1 diabetes.)

Example problem case 2

Problem Case:

The practice has recently taken over the list of a single-handed practice of a GP who has retired. He had a large number of patients with diabetes because of the ethnic mix in his practice. His patients are used to attending the doctor for all their care and are resisting attending the practice diabetic clinic run by two nurses with specialist qualifications in diabetes.

Table 5.1:   Role and responsibilities checklist – *for each task tick the box for each team member who has a role or responsibility – then note your role and responsibilities for the task*

Completed by: _____

| Task | Primary care team member | | | | | | | What are your roles and your responsibilities? |
	Doctor	Practice nurse	District nurse	Reception team	Practice manager	Podiatrist	Other	
Identifying patients who should be included on the register	✔	✔	✔	✔	✔	✔	✔	*e.g. Making sure that people suspected, but not confirmed, of having the condition are **not** included on the register*
Task 2								
Task 3								
Task 4								
Task 5								

Who do you need in your team?

You might want a team that includes:

Practice nurses
GPs
Clerical staff
Patients and carers
District nurses
Pharmacists
Local influential community leaders
Practice manager
Health visitors
Podiatrists
Dietitians
Optometrists.

Where you are now

The practice has invited all the patients who have been taken on to their list to attend a new patient screening medical with the nurses. Very few of them attend. A search of the medical records as they are summarised yields a large number of people with diabetes who have been specifically invited to have a check on their diabetes. The patients continue to turn up to see the GPs with queries about their treatment, to have their feet looked at, with infections, etc. and there is no systematic care. Efforts to transfer the care to the practice diabetic clinic are not productive. Patients either do not make the appointment on their way out from the GP or waste the appointment time by failing to attend.

What you do next

This might include.

- Talking to community leaders to try to discover why there is such resistance to the change from GP opportunistic care to systematic nurse-led care.
- Engaging with a few articulate patients from the new group of patients and asking them to start a patient group for people with diabetes. Help them to set up a meeting on practice premises with a tour of the practice. Arrange talks from specialist nurses and others such as podiatrists, dietitians and optometrists about diabetes and arrange a quiz on diabetes with prizes. Ask them to extend the invitation to all patients with diabetes who attend your practice for their care (a GP from the practice might sign the invitation jointly with the patient group).
- Finding out from the new patients whether they would prefer to attend the nurses' diabetic clinic in groups rather than singly, so that they feel supported by each other.
- The GPs showing their confidence in nurse-led care by personally transferring the patient consulting with a diabetic problem to the specialist nurse. When a medical examination and/or treatment is required (e.g. in infection) the GP makes a point of consulting with the nurse in the nurses' clinic to make sure the patients are aware of the superior service offered by the specialist nurses.

- Using the electronic booking system to make appointments with specialist nurses rather than GPs for patients who declare problems with their diabetes.
- GPs and practice nurses could review their communication skills and attend an updating course if that was appropriate.

What extra resources might this require?

- A senior person willing, able and with time to identify and talk to community leaders. Ability to analyse the information and utilise it to change procedures or approaches.
- A person with the skills and time to facilitate setting up a patient group. A health visitor already known to some of the patient group might be ideal.
- Time to talk to new patients about how they want to contribute their views about services – perhaps by posting them into a suggestion box at reception. Such comments are then collated by the practice secretary and presented at a practice meeting.
- The clinic arrangements for the specialist nurses are modified to allow for a few (depending on demand) free sessions during the day when the doctors are consulting. The patients can then be seen within a reasonable time in the clinic with or without the GP. This should be possible by rearrangement of clinic slots left unused by people who did not attend. If unused, the nurses could use these sessions for extra administration or education time.

The outcomes

- Reduction of resentment and resistance to change with ownership of the new arrangements by the new group of patients with diabetes.
- A gradual transfer of responsibility for care of this group to the specialist nurses.
- Better and more structured management of diabetes.
- Efficient use of practice resources.

How would you demonstrate that you have achieved your outcomes?

An audit of the patients on the diabetic register shows that an increased proportion are receiving structured care with measurement and recording of regular checks.

Problem case exercise

Problem Case:

At a practice meeting, the cost of urine testing strips for albumin:creatinine ratios becomes a hotly debated issue. The GP thinks this test is too expensive for their small practice. He has said that he would refuse to sign prescriptions for urine testing strips that are to be used for patients in general in the nurse's room, rather than just for that patient named on the prescription, as he feels this is unethical. The nurse argues that, as prescriptions for patients with diabetes are free, no-one is disadvantaged and she would be able to carry out tests for microalbuminuria as part of the monitoring for renal disease in diabetes.[1]

(NICE recommends that the albumin:creatinine ratio or the albumin concentration is measured at the annual review for someone with type 2 diabetes. In this scenario, the practice nurse has been on a training course and wants to add this test into the annual review. The practice manager and the GP think the test strips for near-patient testing are very expensive and that the test should be sent off to the laboratory. Some PCOs fund strips for near-patient microalbuminuria detection centrally.)

Who do you need in your team?

Where you are now

What you do next

Continued

What extra resources might this require?

The outcomes

How would you demonstrate that you have achieved your outcomes?

Why the management of diabetes mellitus is important

Diabetes is a chronic, progressive disease that can result in premature death, ill-health and disability. It is the biggest cause of kidney failure, the leading cause of blindness in adults of working age and one of the main causes of lower limb amputation, as well as significantly increasing the risk of coronary heart disease and stroke. The consequences of diabetes can be prevented or delayed by high-quality care and managing the condition in line with the best advice and treatment.

Between 2 and 3% of people of all ages in the UK have type 1 or 2 diabetes.[2] About 200 000 people are thought to have type 1 and more than a million have type 2 diabetes. The lifetime risk for a person living in the UK developing type 2 diabetes is probably greater than 10%.[2]

In the UK, type 2 diabetes is more common in adults of South Asian, African and African-Caribbean origin, Chinese descent and other non-white groups compared with the white population. The prevalence of diabetes mellitus increases with age. As many as one in 20 people over the age of 65 years and one in five over the age of 85 years old in the UK has type 2 diabetes.[2] Diabetes is more common in people from the most deprived sections of the population in the UK, and diabetes complications are several times more likely in people with diabetes from social class V compared to those from social class I.[1,3] Compare the number of people on your diabetes register with local and national figures, taking into consideration your practice characteristics.

What is diabetes?

The World Health Organization (WHO) definition of diabetes is: 'diabetes mellitus describes a metabolic disorder of multiple aetiology characterised by chronic hyper-glycaemia with disturbances of carbohydrate, fat and protein metabolism resulting from defects in insulin secretion, insulin action or both'.[4] One current definition is a fasting plasma glucose of 7.0 mmol/l or above, on two or more occasions. If in doubt, you may need to carry out a glucose tolerance test. Diabetes is confirmed at levels of 11.1 mmol/l or above, two hours after a 75 gram oral glucose load.[5,6]

There are four main sub-categories of diabetes:

1   type 1
2   type 2
3   gestational (carbohydrate intolerance first recognised in pregnancy)
4   other specific types, e.g. drug induced, or secondary to genetic abnormalities.

In people with type 1 diabetes, the pancreas is no longer able to produce insulin because the insulin producing cells (the β-cells) have been destroyed by the body's immune system.

In type 2 diabetes the β-cells are not able to produce enough insulin for the body's needs – and in addition, the majority of people with type 2 diabetes have some degree of resistance to insulin.[3,7] Most of the people with diabetes being managed in general practice will be suffering from type 2 diabetes.

What should you do, when and how?

Initial management of people with newly diagnosed type 2 diabetes[3,6,8]

You might want to write, or update, a checklist so that nothing is forgotten, par-ticularly as you may be part of a team carrying out some of these actions, and the patient may need to attend several times so that everything can be covered. A patient-held record together with a computer template is ideal, but a paper encounter sheet on which all the items are listed and entered as they are completed will help.

Include:

- the history of illness, looking for underlying causes or complications of diabetes
- a simple explanation of diabetes, responding to questions and anxieties from the patient
- a discussion of lifestyle with specific advice about smoking, diet, exercise, and alcohol intake
- an explanation of the practice organisation and the different roles of the primary healthcare team and how to obtain advice as needed
- information about Diabetes UK, how to access it and how it will help.

The examination should include:

- a calculation of body mass index from weight and height measurement
- blood pressure
- a full clinical examination to exclude underlying causes of diabetes such as pancreatic disease, and assess for any existing complications of diabetes.

Investigations may include (the list will vary according to local guidance):

- urinalysis for glucose, ketones and protein (mid-stream urinalysis if micro-albuminuria is detected)
- fasting plasma glucose (as already described above)
- full blood count
- haemoglobin A1c (HbA1c)
- renal profile
- liver function tests
- fasting lipid profile
- thyroid function tests.

Initial management should include:

- referral to a diabetes specialist if the patient is unwell (e.g. has marked recent weight loss), if there is ketonuria or if the blood glucose concentration is over 20 mmol/l. If the patient is reasonably well you might give a three-month trial of dietary treatment
- give each patient with diabetes a named contact from within the practice team
- initial dietary assessment and advice
- referral to dietitian or member of the specialist diabetes team such as community diabetes educator if indicated (and if available)
- referral to podiatrist or chiropodist, and optometrist if necessary
- discussion and agreement of individualised management plan with targets as appropriate: including change to a healthy balanced diet, restriction of refined sugars and alcohol, increasing exercise, stopping smoking – as appropriate
- making follow-up appointments
- entering the patient on practice diabetes register and recall system.

Continuing management of patients with type 2 diabetes[9]

There are two main aims of treatment for diabetes.

1   To allow as normal a daily life as possible without symptoms whilst at the same time avoiding acute complications such as ketoacidosis, hypoglycaemia and infection.

2   To prevent or delay the long-term specific complications of diabetes including microangiopathy (retinopathy, nephropathy), cataract and neuropathy and to decrease the excess morbidity and mortality from cardiovascular disease.[10]

What are the outcomes?

A key outcome measure of good diabetes management is blood glucose control, as measured by how low the levels are of glycated haemoglobin (HbA1c). This indicates the quality of blood glucose control over the preceding two to three months. The target should reflect individual circumstances, aiming between 6.5 and 7.5%.[11]

Other helpful outcome measures include pre- and post-meal blood glucose levels, the extent to which acute episodes of hypoglycaemia and hyperglycaemia are prevented, and reduction in adverse risk factors such as raised blood pressure, smoking, obesity and dyslipidaemia.[10]

You may want to establish follow-up routines for those diagnosed with gestational diabetes as some of them will develop full diabetes. Children and teenagers are usually cared for by secondary care. You will need procedures to add teenagers reaching their 17th birthday by (and after) April 2005 to your diabetes register.

The review of patients with type 2 diabetes will include the indicators covered by the quality and outcomes indicators of the GMS contract (*see* Table 5.2) and are covered in more detail in *Diabetes Matters in Primary Care*.[7] Patients can monitor many of these indicators themselves, e.g. their weight, smoking status, or self-taken blood pressure, and can record information such as the results of their blood tests and when they had retinal screening. This information can then easily be entered into their electronic medical record at their review appointment (until patients are able to carry smart cards with this information).

Table 5.2:   Quality and outcomes measures for diabetes mellitus[12]

Criteria		Maximum threshold (minimum 25%) (%)	Points
DM1	The practice can produce a register of all patients over 17 years of age with diabetes mellitus	Compatible with expected prevalence	6
DM2	Percentage of patients on the diabetic register whose notes record BMI in the previous 15 months	90	3
DM3	Percentage of patients on the diabetic register in whom there is a record of smoking status in the previous 15 months except those who have never smoked where smoking status should be recorded once	90	3
DM4	Percentage of patients on the diabetic register who smoke and whose notes contain a record that smoking cessation advice has been offered in the last 15 months	90	5
DM5	Percentage of patients on the diabetic register who have a record of HbA1c or equivalent in the previous 15 months	90	3

Continued

Table 5.2   *Continued*

Criteria		Maximum threshold (minimum 25%) (%)	Points
DM6	Percentage of patients on the diabetic register in whom the last HbA1c is 7.4 or less (or equivalent test/reference range depending on local laboratory) in last 15 months	50	16
DM7	Percentage of patients on the diabetic register in whom the last HbA1c is 10 or less (or equivalent test/reference range depending on local laboratory) in last 15 months	85	11
DM8	Percentage of patients on the diabetic register who have a record of retinal screening in the previous 15 months	90	5
DM9	Percentage of patients on the diabetic register with a record of presence or absence of peripheral pulses in the previous 15 months	90	3
DM10	Percentage of patients on the diabetic register with a record of neuropathy testing in the previous 15 months	90	3
DM11	Percentage of patients on the diabetic register who have a record of the blood pressure in the past 15 months	90	3
DM12	Percentage of patients on the diabetic register in whom the last blood pressure is 145/85 or less	55	17
DM13	Percentage of patients on the diabetic register who have a record of microalbuminuria testing in the previous 15 months (except patients with proteinuria)	90%	3
DM14	Percentage of patients on the diabetic register who have a record of serum creatinine testing in the previous 15 months	90	3
DM15	Percentage of patients on the diabetic register with proteinuria or microalbuminuria who are treated with ACE inhibitors (or A2 antagonists)	70	3
DM16	Percentage of patients on the diabetic register who have a record of total cholesterol in the previous 15 months	90	3
DM17	Percentage of patients on the diabetic register whose last measured total cholesterol within previous 15 months is 5 or less	60	6
DM18	Percentage of patients on the diabetic register who have had influenza immunisation in the preceding 1 September to 31 March	85	3

Sixty five per cent of the total points are available for the overlapping areas for diabetes, coronary heart disease, heart failure, hypertension and stroke. Maximising the indicators from managing diabetes will benefit patients in other domains.

Some of the information will come from secondary care when tests are carried out there. Set up procedures to record this information in the electronic medical record so that tests are not repeated unnecessarily and uneconomically.

What are the challenges?

- People with type 2 diabetes may mistakenly believe that their condition is trivial because they have no symptoms when they are first identified as having diabetes.
- People faced with long-term disabilities or disease take time to accept the situation. It is like a bereavement – the loss of previous good health – and they may deny the need for constant vigilance about their condition at first. The lifestyle changes required are often significant and patients may resist change.
- Management of your appointment system may be less than optimal. For example, patients may attend for a review appointment when test results are not yet available, so no decisions on future management can be made.
- A lack of resources may make some of the monitoring activity difficult. There is a shortage of dietitians, podiatrists, and nurses trained in diabetes. Testing for microalbuminuria is expensive, and retinal screening may not be accessible to all.

What can you do to make it more likely that you will succeed?

- Give patients simple written information leaflets about diabetes, dietary advice, etc. (so long as they are literate) as well as the contact details of Diabetes UK.
- Re-iterate the advice you give and be patient with those who take time to accept their illness.
- Patients living with long-term medical conditions such as diabetes can be helped by the expert patient programme. Patients who have been through the programme then act as tutors for other patients. The programme covers confidence in accessing services, knowing how to act upon symptoms, dealing with acute attacks or exacerbations of the disease, making the most effective use of medication and treatment, and understanding the implications of advice from professionals.[3,11,13]
- Nominate team members to be responsible for specific tasks with deputies for when they are away, e.g. to record test results or retinal screening results from letters coming in to the practice, or to contact patients who need a review appointment.
- Make contact with diabetes clinic staff in secondary care so that information can be easily transferred in both directions to prevent gaps and duplications. Consider establishing patient-held records.
- Ensure that instructions are explicit, e.g. arrange blood testing for patients one week before their appointment in the diabetic clinic.
- Access interpreters and link workers as appropriate for people who require additional services to increase their understanding and concordance.
- Invest in further nurse training, e.g. a short course or a diploma in diabetic nursing.

Further reading

Chambers R, Stead J and Wakley G (2001) *Diabetes Matters in Primary Care.* Radcliffe Medical Press, Oxford.

References

1 National Institute for Clinical Excellence (2004) *Management of Type 2 Diabetes: renal disease – prevention and early management.* NICE, London. www.nice.org.uk/page.aspx?o= 27964

   Other NICE guidelines are:
   • Blood pressure and lipids: www.nice.org.uk/
   • Footcare: www.nice.org.uk/
   • Blood glucose levels: www.nice.org.uk/
   • Retinopathy: www.nice.org.uk/

2 Williams R and Farrar H (2004) Diabetes Mellitus. In: Stevens A *et al.* (eds) *Health Care Needs Assessment: the epidemiologically based needs assessment reviews,* Volume 1 (2e). Radcliffe Publishing. Oxford. www.radcliffe-oxford.com

3 NHS Executive (2001) *National Service Framework for Diabetes.* Department of Health, London. www.dh.gov.uk/assetRoot/04/05/89/38/04058938.pdf

4 World Health Organization (1999) *Definition, Diagnosis and Classification of Diabetes Mellitus and its Complications – Part 1: diagnosis and classification of diabetes mellitus.* World Health Organization, Geneva. www.diabetes.org.uk/infocentre/carerec/diagnosi.doc

5 Godlee F (ed.) (2004) *Clinical Evidence Concise. Issue 11.* BMJ Publishing Group, London. www.clinicalevidence.com

6 Diabetes UK (1997) *Recommendations for the Management of Diabetes in Primary Care.* Diabetes UK, London. www.diabetes.org.uk

7 Chambers R, Stead J and Wakley G (2001) *Diabetes Matters in Primary Care.* Radcliffe Medical Press, Oxford.

8 Smith S (2003) Newly diagnosed type 2 diabetes mellitus. 10-minute consultation. *BMJ.* **326**: 1371. www.bmj.com

9 Foord-Kelcey G (ed.) (2004) Management of diabetes. *Guidelines* **23**: 219–47. www. eguidelines.co.uk

10 Albert KG (1992) Good control or a happy life? In: Lewin I and Seymour C (1992) *Current Themes in Diabetes Care.* Royal College of Physicians, London.

11 National Institute for Clinical Excellence (NICE) (2003) *Guidance on the Use of Patient-education Models for Diabetes.* Technology appraisal guidance 60. NICE, London. www.nice.org.uk/page.aspx?o=68328

12 General Practitioners Committee/The NHS Confederation (2003) *New GMS Contract. Investing in General Practice.* British Medical Association, London.

13 Department of Health (2001) *The Expert Patient: a new approach to chronic disease management in the 21st century.* Department of Health, London. www.dh.gov.uk

6

Hypertension

To explore how your primary care team might work together to improve the management of patients with hypertension you can review a case (or cases) with which your team has been involved. You may prefer to use the two example cases at the start of this chapter. Read through them quickly before working on the problem case exercise (*see* page 84), or just photocopy Table 1.1 on page 7 to develop your own problem case. Include in your team people who will join in the problem-based learning discussion and be part of the solutions.

If you feel that you have insufficient knowledge to guide you in completing the problem-based learning, use the summary about hypertension in the second part of this chapter and follow up the references if you need to learn more.

Example problem case 1

> **Problem Case:**
>
> An audit by the practice manager shows that 38% of patients on the hypertensive register have not been reviewed in the last nine months.

Who do you need in your team?

You might want a team that includes:

Carer/patient/pharmacist requesting regular repeat medication
Reception staff doing repeat prescriptions
Practice manager
Staff responsible for recalling patients
Nurses and doctors seeing patients for other conditions.

Where you are now

On examining the audit figures more closely it becomes apparent that this is because patients have not requested their medication, so that a recall for review has not been triggered.

What you do next

This might include.

- Obtaining the views of patients on hypertensive medication and reasons why they did not request medication.
- Looking at the literature about why people do not take anti-hypertensive medication.
- Producing or adapting a patient resource pack about hypertension. Pilot it with patients and staff. Re-write it taking their feedback into account.
- Arranging for all staff to attend a meeting so that they understand the need for concordance and rehearse explaining the reasons for controlling blood pressure with patients, using case scenarios.
- Arranging health promotion activities for patients around the theme of hypertension and prevention of arteriosclerosis.
- Putting in place a regular audit to pick up people on the register who have not been reviewed and inviting them for a health check.
- Completing Table 6.1.

What extra resources might this require?

- Staff time for sending out questionnaires and collating the information.
- Time to look at and evaluate the literature.
- Time and costs of making a patient resource pack, piloting it and re-writing it.
- Time and resources for a staff meeting.
- Input from health promotion and provision of premises, etc. for health promotion activities.
- Clerical time for audit.
- Clerical time, stationery and postage costs for invitations.

The outcomes

The outcomes might include 90% of patients on the hypertension register have a recorded blood pressure reading in the last nine months.

How would you demonstrate that you have achieved your outcomes?

Repeat audit at intervals to measure progress towards the target.

Example problem case 2

> **Problem Case:**
>
> The practice recently appointed two of the reception staff as healthcare assistants (HCAs). Amongst their responsibilities is blood pressure recording. At a practice meeting one of the GPs complains that he is seeing large numbers of people for review of raised readings. He then takes the blood pressure, considers it within normal limits and tells the patients that the readings are fine – no treatment, or no change of treatment, is necessary.

Table 6.1: Role and responsibilities checklist – *for each task tick the box for each team member who has a role or responsibility – then note your role and responsibilities for the task*

Completed by: _____

| Task | Primary care team member | | | | | | | What are your roles and your responsibilities? |
	Doctor	Practice nurse	HCA	Reception team	Practice manager	Podiatrist	Other	
Identifying patients who should be included on the register	✔	✔	✔	✔	✔	✔	✔	*e.g. Making sure that people suspected, but not confirmed, of having the condition are **not** included on the register*
Task 2								
Task 3								
Task 4								
Task 5								

Who do you need in your team?

You might want a team that includes:

GPs
Practice nurses
Healthcare assistants
Practice manager
Patient.

Where you are now

Management issues might include.

- How often does this occur (i.e. is it significant enough to matter)?
- Is this *both* healthcare assistants (HCAs) or only one of them?
- Is it a training/education issue (for either GP or HCA)?
- Is it a resistance to change issue (from GP, practice nurse, HCA or patients)?
- Is it a problem with poor, or inadequately maintained or calibrated, equipment?

Healthcare assistant issues might include.

- Lack of confidence in their competence to do the task.
- Are others in the team (e.g. practice nurse, GP) supporting them in their new role?
- Is the referral protocol too restrictive?

Practice nurse issues might include.

- Resentment at removal of simpler tasks that allowed her to catch up during clinics.
- Lack of time to advise or supervise the HCA.
- Lack of knowledge or skills to train or supervise the HCA correctly.
- Resistance to change.

GP issues might include.

- Resistance to change.
- Lack of agreement with the protocol.
- Individual variation of interpretation of the significance of blood pressure readings.
- Lack of knowledge or skills.

What you do next

This might include.

- Obtaining the views of all involved about the perceived advantages or disadvantages of the present system, including patient views.
- Carrying out an education campaign about blood pressure with patients.
- Encouraging home recording of blood pressures by patients requiring monitoring.
- Comparing the blood pressure readings taken by the HCA and the GPs.
- Auditing the standards of technique of all those taking blood pressures.
- Checking all blood pressure equipment for reliability and accuracy.
- Re-examining the protocol for referral from the HCA in a practice meeting.

What extra resources might this require?

- Time and resources for patient education.
- Replacement of inadequate blood pressure equipment.
- Arrangements for regular calibration of devices in use.

The outcomes

- Improved understanding of blood pressure recording variations by team members and patients.
- A move towards increased home recording of blood pressures by patients requiring monitoring.
- Improved standards of blood pressure recording techniques.
- A more useful protocol for referral of raised blood pressure recordings from the HCA.

How would you demonstrate that you have achieved your outcomes?

- Improved concordance with treatment objectives.
- Improved feedback from patients and staff.
- Fewer discordant blood pressure readings by different observers.

Problem case exercise

Problem Case:

A significant event audit is presented at a practice meeting. A patient who was being treated for hypertension with bendroflumethiazide for several years had been admitted to hospital following a road traffic accident and was found to have diabetes. His medical record does not include any blood or urine tests. The practice team wants to ensure that this lack of care or recording does not occur again.

Who do you need in your team?

Where you are now

What you do next

Continued

What extra resources might this require?

The outcomes

How would you demonstrate that you have achieved your outcomes?

Why controlling hypertension is important

Systolic and diastolic pressures are continuously related to the risk of developing cardiovascular disease and the risk extends into the range usually regarded as 'normal' blood pressures. In controlled trials over three to five years, drug treatment for hypertension prevents cardiovascular complications, but little is known about long-term prognosis. A follow-up study of 20 to 22 years showed that treated males with hypertension had significantly increased mortality, especially from coronary heart disease compared with males without hypertension, from the same population.[1] The high incidence of coronary heart disease was related to organ damage, smoking and cholesterol levels at the time of entry to the study. So, you should not look at levels of blood pressure in isolation but at whole people and their risk factors. Reducing blood pressure helps to prevent stroke, but other risk factors (e.g. smoking, cholesterol levels) are likely to be more important in preventing other cardiovascular adverse events.

What is hypertension?

Definitions for 'hypertension' vary according to the country and population and have changed over time.[2] The *National Service Framework for Coronary Heart Disease* defines hypertension as:[3]

'a sustained systolic blood pressure of 140 mmHg (mercury) or more, or a diastolic blood pressure of 85 mmHg or more'

and treatment at lower limits for those who have **other risk factors**:

'sustained systolic pressure of 140–159 mmHg or diastolic pressures of 85–99 mmHg'

Other risk factors include:

1   evidence of established cardiovascular disease
2   diabetes
3   a ten-year risk of cardiovascular disease of more than 15% using one of the coronary heart disease risk charts[4]
4   the presence of target organ damage.

The British Hypertension Society Guidelines have modified their categories (*see* Table 6.2) to bring them into line with European standards.[5]

Table 6.2:   British Hypertension Society categories of hypertension

Category	Systolic blood pressure, mmHg	Diastolic blood pressure, mmHg
Optimal blood pressure	< 120	< 80
Normal blood pressure	< 130	< 85
High–normal blood pressure	130–139	85–89
Grade 1 hypertension (mild)	140–159	90–99
Grade 2 hypertension (moderate)	160–179	100–109
Grade 3 hypertension (severe)	> 180	> 110
Isolated systolic hypertension (Grade 1)	140–159	< 90
Isolated systolic hypertension (Grade 2)	> 160	< 90

National surveys show that there is a substantial under-diagnosis, under-treatment and poor rates of blood pressure control in the UK.[5]

What should you do, when and how?

Guidelines for the assessment and treatment of patients with hypertension should be up to date and accessible to all clinical staff, such as healthcare assistants, nurses and doctors. The British Hypertension Society guidelines appear in *Guidelines* or on the eguidelines website.[6]

Measure and record

Measure blood pressures in all patients every five years and annually in those patients who have raised readings. Base your confirmation of hypertension on readings from the initial visit plus two follow-up visits with at least two readings at each visit. Use standardised methods for recording blood pressures (*see* Box 6.1).

Box 6.1:   Measuring blood pressure

- Use a properly maintained, calibrated and validated device
- Measure sitting blood pressure routinely: standing blood pressure should be recorded at the initial estimation in the elderly and patients with diabetes
- Remove tight clothing, support the arm at heart level, ensure the hand is relaxed and avoid talking during the measurement procedure
- Use a cuff of appropriate size (large size for large arms)
- If not using electronic machine, lower pressure slowly (2 mm/second), read blood pressure to the nearest 2 mmHg, measure diastolic as disappearance of sounds (phase V)
- Take the mean of at least two readings. More recordings are needed if you find marked differences between initial measurements
- Do not treat on the basis of an isolated reading. Take at least three readings on separate occasions

For full details of methods and suitable equipment look at the British Hypertension Society website.[5]

Investigate for remedial conditions

You want to establish if the patient has any:

- underlying cause for hypertension (*see* Table 6.3)
- other risk factors present (smoking, obesity, diabetes, etc.)
- complications are already present (e.g. previous stroke)
- end-organ damage (e.g. left ventricular hypertrophy)
- other conditions that might affect treatment (e.g. asthma, preventing the use of beta-blocker drugs).

History and examination will reveal most of these factors. A list of investigations that might help to identify these conditions might include:

- urine test strip for blood and protein
- blood electrolytes and creatinine

Table 6.3:   Underlying causes for hypertension (present in about 5–10% of cases)[7]

Cause	What to look for
Drug induced	non-steroidal anti-inflammatory drugs, corticosteroids, combined oral contraceptives, cyclosporin, erythropoietin
Endocrine	
primary aldosteronism	tetany, muscle weakness, polyuria, hypokalaemia
Cushing's syndrome	truncal obesity, striae, etc.
phaeochromocytoma	intermittent high blood pressure, sweating attacks, palpitations
acromegaly	enlargement of hands and feet, coarsening of facial features, visual field loss, etc.
Vascular	
coarctation of aorta	delayed or weak femoral pulses
renal artery stenosis	peripheral vascular disease, abdominal bruit
Renal	
chronic pyelonephritis	history of recurrent infections
diabetic nephropathy	microalbuminuria or proteinuria
glomerulonephritis	microscopic haematuria
obstructive uropathy	abdominal or flank mass
polycystic kidneys	abdominal or flank mass, microscopic haematuria, family history
Connective tissue disorders	symptoms or signs of scleroderma, systemic lupus erythematosis, polyarteritis nodosa, retroperitoneal fibrosis

- fasting blood glucose
- fasting lipid profile, including ratio of serum total cholesterol to high density lipoprotein (HDL) cholesterol
- electrocardiogram.

The European Society of Hypertension guidelines also recommend echocardiography as a routine investigation to detect ischaemia, conduction defects and arrhythmias.[7] However, this may not be practicable in your area if long waiting lists for echo-cardiography exist. You might need to give priority to people with severe disease or clinical suspicion of heart failure.

You should refer patients to secondary care when they have:

- an underlying cause as they will require specialist investigations
- very high blood pressure levels (more than 220/120 mmHg), accelerated rises (malignant hypertension) or impending complications
- treatment difficulties, e.g. poor control on three medications, side-effects or contraindications to medication
- special problems, e.g. unusually variable levels, pregnancy.

Treat energetically

Encourage lifestyle interventions (*see* Table 6.4) in patients who have mild hyper-tension but no target organ damage or cardiovascular complications. Reassess after

Table 6.4:   Non-drug treatments of hypertension[8]

To lower blood pressure	To reduce the risk of cardiovascular disease
Weight reduction	Stop smoking
Take dynamic exercise, such as brisk walking (rather than isometric exercise, such as weight training)	Reduce saturated fat in the diet and replace it with polyunsaturated or monounsaturated fat
Limit alcohol to less than 21 units (men) or 15 units (women) per week	Increase the intake of oily fish
Reduce added salt, or avoid salty food	
Increase the intake of fruit and vegetables and decrease the saturated and total fat intake	

four to six months. Introduce these interventions at the same time as medication in patients when drug treatment is indicated. Evidence about changing behaviour shows that it *is* worth making the effort to advise people about lifestyle changes.[8] Lifestyle changes can make a substantial impact on risk factors and even small changes in weight can reduce blood pressure readings – blood pressure falls by 2.5/1.5 mmHg for each kilogram of weight loss.

The hypertension optimal treatment (HOT)[9] trial suggested that the optimal blood pressure for reduction of cardiovascular events was 139/83 mmHg. The numbers in this trial were not large and the group whose blood pressure was below 150/90 mmHg had no obvious disadvantages. Patients with diabetes had greater lowering of their risk if their diastolic blood pressure was kept below 80 mmHg. Discuss the optimal treatment with each patient as not everyone will be willing or able to achieve these targets. Record your discussion to back up any claim for exemption from your targets in the quality and outcomes framework.

Anti-hypertensive drug therapy

Three long-term, double blind studies compared the major classes of anti-hypertensive drugs and found no consistent or important differences in efficacy, side-effects or quality of life.[5] There were differences between the classes of drugs related to ethnic group and age. Treatment trials with beta blockers or thiazides provide most of the evidence about benefits of blood pressure lowering for reduction of cardiovascular risk. Trials of medication for hypertension have some limitations. Most patients in the trials had high additional risk factors such as diabetes and compliance with treatment in trials is much higher than in clinical practice. These controlled randomised trials lasted for four to five years, whereas life expectancy in middle-aged people with hypertension is 20 to 30 years.[5] Consider individual patient variations when deciding on which treatment to choose.[4–8]

Tailor the drug regimen to suit the patient whenever possible. If there are no indications to direct the first choice to specific drugs, then a low dose of a thiazide, e.g. bendroflumethiazide 2.5 mg or hydrochlorthiazide 25 mg, is cost effective. The dose-response curve for thiazides shows that increasing the dose does not increase efficacy, so change the type of medication, or add in another, if there is a poor response. Unless very urgent, change therapy only after an interval of about four weeks. Always check first that the patient is taking his or her medication. Concordance, not compliance, is important in treating a condition in which patients may feel less well on treatment than without (*see* page 172).

It is reasonable to start treatment either with a low dose of a single agent or with a low dose combination of two agents.[5-7] If you choose low-dose single agent therapy and blood pressure control is not achieved, the next step is to switch to a low dose of a different agent. Alternatively, you could increase the dose of the first preparation chosen (with a greater possibility of causing adverse effects) or move to combination therapy. If you started with a low-dose combination, you can use a higher dose combination or add a low dose of a third medication.

Many patients will need more than one type of therapy to achieve reduction of blood pressure to target levels. Try to give as few drugs as possible and preferably in a single daily dose. Multiple dosing increases the risk of forgotten tablets. Check for interactions between drugs before combining.

Fixed-dose combinations may be sensible and convenient once the patient is happy with the medication and well controlled, provided there are no major cost implications. Beware of unfamiliar drug combinations that may contain the same class of drug as already being prescribed singly. The Prodigy guideline on hypertension contains detailed lists of recommended medication for treatment of hypertension.[10]

Special groups of patients with hypertension

Ethnic groups

Patients of Asian origin with hypertension are more at risk of diabetes and coronary artery disease. Use thiazides with caution as they can worsen glucose intolerance. Patients of African-Caribbean origin seem to respond less well to beta-blockers and ACE inhibitors and achieve better control on thiazide and calcium channel antagonists.[11]

Older people

Hypertension, especially isolated systolic hypertension (160 mmHg systolic with a diastolic of less than 90 mmHg) is found in more than half of those over 60 years. Over 60-year olds with hypertension have a higher risk of cardiovascular complications than younger people. Women over the age of 70 years have a higher risk of cardiovascular disease, particularly of stroke, than men of that age. Treatment, continued to at least the age of 80 years, has been shown to reduce the risks.[5] Thiazides are the first choice for drug treatment or dihydropyridine calcium antagonists if thiazides are contraindicated, not tolerated or are ineffective.

Patients with diabetes

Comparative trials suggest that ACE inhibitors are better than calcium channel antagonists in preventing cardiovascular events.[8] As far as possible levels of blood pressure in people with diabetes should be controlled to below 140/80 mmHg.

Malignant hypertension

This is an emergency, fortunately rare, with a very poor outcome if left untreated. Even when treated a high proportion go on to develop strokes or renal failure. The diagnostic criteria are a diastolic blood pressure of over 120 mmHg together with advanced hypertensive retinopathy (haemorrhages and exudates, with or without papilloedema). It is more common in smokers and people of African-Caribbean origin. Recommended treatment includes a reduction in blood pressure over about one week (to avoid precipitating a stroke by too rapid a reduction). You will probably want to seek specialist help especially as secondary hypertension is more common in this group than in non-malignant hypertension and patients will require investigation to exclude a precipitating cause.

Monitor

The frequency of follow-up visits will depend on the overall risk category of the patient, as well as on the level of blood pressure. Once the target level of blood pressure has been reached and other risk factors have been controlled or excluded, agree a follow-up regime with the patient. Some patients are happy to monitor their own blood pressure at home (with a suitable machine) and can be seen less often. If a stabilised patient expresses undue anxiety about lengthening the interval between checks to six-monthly, this is an opportunity to correct any misconceptions about the aims of treatment.

Patients not on drug treatment should understand the need for monitoring and follow-up and for periodic reconsideration of the need for drug treatment.

In more complex cases, patients should be seen at more frequent intervals. If the therapeutic goals, including the control of blood pressure, have not been reached within six months, consider referral to a specialist in hypertension.

Anti-hypertensive therapy is generally for life. Stopping treatment in patients who have been correctly diagnosed as hypertensive is usually followed, sooner or later, by the return of blood pressure to pre-treatment levels. Nevertheless, after prolonged blood pressure control, you may be able to gradually reduce the dose or number of drugs used, particularly among patients who have made great strides in observing lifestyle (non-drug) measures. Keep monitoring carefully to ensure that levels do not climb steadily upwards with a reduction in medication, or with an increase in weight with increasing age. Remain alert to any incipient additional risk factors.

What are the outcomes?

You should aim to achieve the following.

1 Increase the proportion of patients who have recorded blood pressures.
2 Increase the proportion of patients who understand the preventive reasons for blood pressure recording and that hypertension does not give symptoms.
3 Provide education about the use of non-pharmacological interventions for patients with risk factors for hypertension, e.g. high-normal blood pressure, and those who have established hypertension.
4 Improve the assessment of those with hypertension.
5 Increase the percentage of patients whose hypertension is controlled.

These aims are recognised in the quality and outcomes framework.

Table 6.5:　Quality and outcomes measures for hypertension

Criteria	Maximum thresholds (minimum 25%) (%)	Points
A register of all patients with a blood pressure over a systolic of 160 and a diastolic of 100 mmHg measured according to the British Hypertension Society Guidelines	Practice prevalence in line with national/local prevalence figures	9
Percentage of patients over 45 years of age screened for hypertension	75	15
Percentage of patients who have their smoking status recorded in the last 15 months	90	10
Percentage of patients who smoke who have been offered smoking cessation advice in the last 15 months	90	10
Percentage of patients on the hypertension register who have had a blood pressure measurement in the last nine months	90	20
Percentage of patients who have a blood pressure on treatment of less than that recommended by the British Hypertension Society Guidelines (BP150/90) in the last 15 months	70	19

Quality indicators in hypertension

A total of 105 points are available for hypertension management (*see* Table 6.5). A further 53 points can be found in the management of blood pressure in the diabetes, coronary heart disease and stroke indicator sets. Organisational points for screening the practice population for hypertension add another 15 points.

　　Patients can be excluded from these targets if they:

- refuse, or fail to attend, at least three invitations in the last 12 months
- refuse to allow their blood pressure to be measured
- have a condition that renders hypertension management irrelevant, e.g. they are terminally ill
- cannot tolerate, or have contraindications to, medication to control the hypertension
- have been diagnosed with hypertension for less than nine months.

What are the challenges?

- Keeping up to date with a rapidly changing evidence base and balancing the differing recommendations.
- Gaining access to the hard-to-reach groups, e.g. males between 20 and 50 years of age.
- Educating people so that they understand why they should make lifestyle changes or take medication when they felt perfectly well before.

- Supporting people who are having difficulties making lifestyle changes or coping with adverse effects of medication.

What can you do to make it more likely that you will succeed?

- Take blood pressure measurement to the patients. Provide many opportunities for measurement, e.g. at the pharmacy, in the pub, at social events. Think about how you might involve people in taking their own blood pressure. You might provide lists of approved measuring devices and sources from which patients might purchase them (pharmacies, mail order, websites). You might invest in a static self-administered machine (connected to a computer or printing out the result) so that patients can take their blood pressure before going in to see the health professional.
- Educate the practice population about hypertension and treatment options.
- Use computerised prompts to check blood pressure at suitable intervals.
- Set up recall systems with a patient register.

Further reading

Chambers R, Wakley G and Iqbal Z (2001) *Cardiovascular Disease Matters in Primary Care.* Radcliffe Medical Press, Oxford.

Wakley G, Chambers R and Ellis S (2004) *Demonstrating Your Competence 3: cardiovascular and neurological conditions.* Radcliffe Publishing, Oxford.

References

1   Anderson OK, Almgreen T, Persoson B *et al.* (1998) Survival after treated hypertension. *BMJ.* **317**: 167–71.

2   Fahey TP and Peters TJ (1996) What constitutes controlled hypertension? Patient based comparison of hypertension guidelines. *BMJ.* **313**: 93–6.

3   NHS Executive (2000) *National Service Framework for Coronary Heart Disease.* Department of Health, London. www.dh.gov.uk/assetRoot/04/04/90/70/04049070.pdf

4   Joint Formulary Committee (2003) *British National Formulary.* British Medical Association and Royal Pharmaceutical Society, London. www.bnf.org

5   Williams B, Poulter NR, Brown MJ *et al.* (2004) Guidelines for management of hypertension: report of the fourth working party of the British Hypertension Society, 2004 – BHS IV. *Journal of Human Hypertension.* **18**: 139–85. www.hyp.ac.uk/bhs/pdfs/BHS_IV_Guidelines.pdf

6   Foord-Kelcey G (ed.) (2004) *Guidelines Volume 23.* Medenium Group Publishing Ltd, Berkhamsted. www.eguidelines.co.uk

7   Guidelines Committee (2003) European Society of Hypertension – European Society of Cardiology guidelines for the management of arterial hypertension. *Journal of Hypertension.* **21(6)**: 1011–53.

8   Godlee F (ed.) (2004) *Clinical Evidence*. BMJ Publishing Group, London. www.clinicalevidence.com

9   Hypertension Optimal Treatment Study Group (1998) Effects of intensive blood-pressure lowering and low-dose aspirin in patients with hypertension: principal results of the hypertension optimal treatment (HOT) randomized trial. *Lancet*. **351**: 1755–62.

10 www.prodigy.nhs.uk

11 Lip GYH, O'Brien E and Beevers G (eds) (2000) *ABC of Hypertension* (4e). BMJ Publications, London.

7

Hypothyroid disease

To explore how your primary care team might work together to improve the management of patients with hypothyroidism you can review a case (or cases) with which your team has been involved. You may prefer to use the two example cases at the start of this chapter. Read through them quickly before working on the problem case exercise (*see* page 100), or just photocopy Table 1.1 on page 7 to develop your own problem case. Include in your team people who will join in the problem-based learning discussion and be part of the solutions.

If you feel that you have insufficient knowledge to guide you in completing the problem-based learning, use the summary about hypothyroidism in the second part of this chapter and follow up the references if you need to learn more.

Example problem case 1

Problem Case:

The practice manager brings the results of the recent search for data on hypothyroid monitoring to the attention of the practice. The results six months ago gave grounds for optimism, but the latest percentages are lower.

Who do you need in your team?

You might want a team that includes:

Reception staff
Practice manager
Phlebotomists
Practice nurses
District nurses
GPs
Patients and carers
Pharmacists
Nursing-home staff.

Where you are now

When the hypothyroid disease register was set up all patients on levothyroxine were included. It had been decided that people suspected of having hypothyroidism would not be entered under the related Read code until the diagnosis had been confirmed biochemically. It appears that the diagnosis of acquired hypothyroidism is not being coded when it is confirmed, nor are the tests being coded when completed.

What you do next

A working group of those involved propose that:

- the clinician responsible for looking at the biochemical confirmation of the condition (e.g. GP or practice nurse) is responsible for coding the diagnosis, so that this can be picked up by the software to compile the register
- named individuals, with a named deputy, will be responsible for entering the code for a thyroid function test when the test results are received, not entering it as free text. This ensures that tests taken at home are included in the system
- the software sets an automatic annual recall date for the next test at the same time as this test result is entered, but this date can be altered so that testing can be more frequent if required. The date is to appear on the righthand side of the repeat prescription slip, so that patients and staff are aware of when it is due
- a patient information sheet is attached to all repeat prescriptions of levothyroxine that explains why testing is necessary
- all patients on amiodarone, lithium and those with a previous history of hyper-thyroidism are recalled for an annual thyroid function test.

You complete Table 7.1.

What extra resources might this require?

- Training in the relevant code-entering procedures for all those involved.
- Time set aside for looking at test results and entering relevant information as codes on the computer system.
- Suitably trained clerical staff code the results marked as normal. Abnormal results are passed to the relevant clinician. Further training expands the system to include other normal results so that clinician time is freed up.
- Finding or preparing a suitable information sheet for patients.

The outcomes

- The register of patients with hypothyroidism is kept up to date.
- Thyroid function tests are coded so that they can be retrieved by software interrogation.
- Patients are recalled for testing at least annually.
- Patients understand why they should attend for monitoring.

How would you demonstrate that you have achieved your outcomes?

- A search of the register after six months shows that the numbers of patients classed as having hypothyroid disease has increased and are at projected levels.

Table 7.1: Role and responsibilities checklist – *for each task tick the box for each team member who has a role or responsibility – then note your role and responsibilities for the task*

Completed by: _____

| Task | Primary care team member | | | | | | | | What are your roles and your responsibilities? |
	Doctor	Practice nurse	District nurse	Reception team	Practice manager	Phlebotomist	Pharmacist	Nursing home staff	
Identifying patients who should be included on the register	✔	✔	✔	✔	✔	✔	✔	✔	e.g. Making sure that people suspected, but not confirmed, of having the condition are **not** included on the register
Recording thyroid function	✔	✔		✔		✔			e.g. Making specific people responsible for coding the test results and entering the date for the next test
Task 3									
Task 4									
Task 5									

- Feedback from patients shows that they like the new clear instructions of when to have another test and understand why the test is needed.
- Thyroid function test monitoring is easy to retrieve by computer search.

Example problem case 2

Problem Case:

Mrs Anxious has made a written complaint about a delayed diagnosis. She has recently been seen at orthopaedic outpatients after a long wait for an appointment, about her increasing difficulty climbing stairs. She has been found to have hypothyroidism and the doctor she saw for her follow-up appointment expressed surprise that she had not been checked for this as she had a history of treatment with radioiodine 12 years previously when she was living in another area.

Who do you need in your team?

You might want a team that includes:

Patients and carers
Practice nurses
GPs
Clerical staff
District nurse
Practice manager
Physiotherapist
Slimming club organisers
Cleaners.

Where you are now

A significant event audit finds that Mrs Anxious always demanded referral to a specialist for any complaint. She had not been followed up after her treatment of hyperthyroidism. It appears this was because she had presented with quite a variety of other complaints since moving to the area and her previous history had been over-looked. She tended to make urgent appointments with whoever was available, be referred to secondary care and no one GP felt responsible for her care or follow-up. Her records contained the information that she had been attending local slimming clubs intermittently trying to lose weight. The practice does not have a system in place for arranging recall for patients who have been treated for hyperthyroidism in the past.

What you do next

This might include.

- Preparing a list of patients who have a history of treatment for hyperthyroidism.[1]
- Arranging an annual recall system for them.[2]

- Preparing an explanatory letter to send to all patients involved about the new arrangements.
- Responding to the complaint according to your complaints procedure, thanking Mrs Anxious for drawing the problem to your attention and explaining what the practice will do to rectify the situation.
- Arranging a clinical meeting at which two reputable local organisations for weight loss will talk about their approaches to weight loss. The practice nurse does a short presentation about the symptoms of hypothyroidism, as well as talking about her approach to weight management. Many of the receptionists are very keen to attend and the practice manager (who also has a personal interest) arranges a 'healthy diet' buffet.

What extra resources might this require?

- The receptionist responsible for searches is given protected time to compile a list of all patients with a coded diagnosis of hyperthyroidism.
- The doctors and nurses agree to add anyone not listed that they discover has a history of treatment for hyperthyroidism.
- The practice secretary who codes the information from hospital letters adds relevant patients to the list proactively.
- Notices are prepared and placed by the reception desk asking people to tell the practice if they have had treatment for thyroid problems in the past.
- The letter is written and the practice cleaners and some patients are asked if they would read and feed back whether it is clear.
- Extra slots are allocated for the phlebotomist to take the annual blood test.

The outcomes

- A comprehensive list of patients requiring follow-up after treatment for hyperthyroidism.
- Regular annual testing of people on this list.
- Early identification of patients developing recurrent hyperthyroidism or a hypothyroid state.
- Greater awareness of patients of the possible longer-term outcomes of their condition.

How would you demonstrate that you have achieved your outcomes?

- Audit the list of patients requiring follow-up after treatment for hyperthyroidism annually to establish the take-up rate for testing.
- A number of patients who have no record of treatment for hyperthyroidism volunteer this information, following the publicity efforts.

Problem case exercise

> **Problem Case:**
>
> Dr Bright brings an observation to a clinical meeting. He says he has started doing a thyroid function test on all new patients found to have raised cholesterol readings and has found two new cases of hypothyroidism. He proposes that this should be standard practice.[3]

Who do you need in your team?

Where you are now

What you do next

What extra resources might this require?

Continued

The outcomes

How would you demonstrate that you have achieved your outcomes?

Why controlling hypothyroidism is important

Hypothyroidism occurs in around four in 1000 women on average, rising to eight in 1000 people over 70 years old. Women are six times more likely to suffer from hypothyroidism than men. Up to 10% of women over 60 years of age have sub-clinical hypothyroidism with moderately raised thyroid stimulating hormone (TSH) and normal levels of thyroid hormone. Significantly higher rates of myocardial infarction and atherosclerosis occur in hypothyroidism. Depression and memory impairment are associated with hypothyroidism.[4]

What is hypothyroidism?

Primary hypothyroidism occurs after destruction of the thyroid gland because of an autoimmune state (i.e. chronic autoimmune thyroiditis) or medical intervention such as surgery, radioiodine or radiation treatment or the side-effects from drugs such as amiodarone or lithium. Secondary hypothyroidism occurs after damage to the pituitary gland or hypothalamus.[4]

The underactivity of the thyroid gland results in reduced levels of the thyroid hormone, thyroxine. The symptoms and signs are a gradual onset of symptoms, increasing lethargy and depression, memory loss and intolerance of the cold. Other symptoms include hair loss, puffy eyes, husky voice, bradycardia, constipation, dizziness, irregular menstruation, infertility, dementia, and delayed relaxation of tendon reflexes.[4,5] A blood test showing results of a TSH over 12 mU/l and a low serum thyroxine (T4 less than 60 nmol/l) confirms the diagnosis. Raised cholesterol levels are also found. In primary hypothyroidism (myxoedema), the thyroid gland may not be palpable and be atrophic, or the patient may have the firm, irregular goitre of Hashimoto's thyroiditis.

What should you do, when and how?

Following treatment for hyperthyroidism

Patients who are treated with radioiodine or have thyroid surgery should be placed on a practice disease register and have their thyroid function tested annually.[2,5] Fifty per cent will become hypothyroid over time and require prescribed thyroxine. There is a 50% relapse rate after stopping carbimazole, so annual follow-up should continue indefinitely for these patients too. They should then be considered for radioiodine or thyroid surgery.

Most people with sub-clinical hypothyroidism do not progress to overt hypothyroidism.[5]

Sub-clinical hypothyroidism

The advice is to simply observe thyroid function over time (e.g. with annual testing of TSH) without treating their sub-clinical state with thyroxine.[5] Research is inconclusive about the benefits of treating sub-clinical hypothyroidism. Treatment can induce hyperthyroidism and reduce bone mass in postmenopausal women and increase the risk of atrial fibrillation, as for overt hyperthyroidism.[5] A consensus statement by the American Association of Clinical Endocrinologists and the Royal College of Physicians recommends that thyroxine therapy is appropriate in patients with a TSH over 10 mU/l, who are the most likely group to progress from sub-clinical to overt hypothyroidism.[5]

Maintenance treatment of hypothyroidism

Levothyroxine is the treatment of choice for treatment for overt hypothyroidism, usually at a dose between 100 to 200 micrograms daily, which can be administered as a single dose.[6] The aim is to achieve a serum TSH within the normal range. A raised free T4 and suppressed TSH indicates overtreatment and is associated with adverse consequences such as an increased risk of developing atrial fibrillation and death from vascular disease, and reduced bone mineral density in postmenopausal women.

What are the outcomes?

The practice reports the number of patients on its hypothyroidism disease register as a proportion of total list size. Check your numbers against prevalence data. You may need to check that those who have a diagnosis have had it confirmed with thyroid function tests, especially those whose diagnosis was made some years ago.

The quality and outcomes framework does not require practices to detect patients at high risk of developing hypothyroidism. Once you have a basic register of all patients with hypothyroidism, consider how you might set up testing for thyroid stimulating hormone by following up annually at-risk patients:

- with a previous history of hyperthyroidism
- who have been treated with partial thyroidectomy or radioactive iodine
- who are taking amiodarone
- who are taking lithium
- with a history of pituitary disease.

Patients with diabetes are at risk of developing hypothyroidism, and a TSH test is recommended as part of the annual diabetes review.

Adding to the register in this way is in line with the consensus statement for management of thyroid disorders and will help to keep your register up to date.[5] The aim of treatment is for test results to show that sufficient thyroxine is circulating and the TSH is within the normal range.

Quality indicators in thyroid monitoring

Although this domain generates the lowest number of points in the clinical section, it should be relatively easy to obtain the maximum number as shown in Table 7.2. As well, remember that scoring points in eight of the ten clinical domains will earn up to 100 extra points for holistic care.

Table 7.2: Quality and outcomes measures for thyroid disease

Criteria	Percentage thresholds (minimum 25%) (%)	Points
The practice can produce a register of patients with hypothyroidism	Compatible with expected prevalence	2
The percentage of patients with a thyroid function test in the last 15 months	90	6

Patients can be excluded from these targets if they are recorded as unsuitable (due to terminal illness, etc.) or have their informed dissent recorded. Do not forget to remove people from the register who move away or die.

What are the challenges?

- Check the numbers on your register against prevalence data. You may need to check that those who have a diagnosis have had it confirmed with thyroid function tests, especially those whose diagnosis was made some years ago. If your numbers are low think how you can identify those you have missed. Mean incidence is 3.5 per 1000 for women and 0.6 per 1000 for men.[5] In a practice of approximately 9000 patients, there will be around 500 and 600 patients taking thyroxine, giving a prevalence of approximately 6%. Hypothyroidism is screened for at birth as part of the Guthrie test. No screening is carried out later as the identification rate is too low to justify a programme.

- With any long-term condition, the risks of failure to take the prescribed medication are considerable, especially as the effects are subtle in the early stages of under-replacement. People miss tablets or fail to take them for a considerable period before clinical effects of hypothyroidism recur.
- Patients may not be monitored because:
    - they do not turn up for the test
    - medication is not renewed and no fail safe mechanism picks this up
    - the practice team continue to prescribe without notifying the patient that testing is required
    - the test is not acted upon because of system failures in the procedure for laboratory reports, e.g. the practice relies on the patient contacting the surgery for the result.

What can you do to make it more likely that you will succeed?

- Ensure that all patients on thyroid replacement therapy are entered on the disease register and that they have had their diagnosis confirmed. Lower than expected numbers should prompt a manual search and prospective recording of all patients seen over a 12- to 24-month period.
- Ensure that all thyroid function tests are coded correctly and acted upon if required.
- Aim for concordance with medication and testing between you and the patient, not compliance (*see* page 172). Ensure that adequate patient education is in place about the necessity for lifelong treatment and accurate monitoring.
- Set up a system to search for all patients with a diagnosis of hypothyroidism at regular intervals, e.g. every three months. Exclude from your search all those who have had a thyroid function test within the last 12 months. Recall those who have not had a test in the last 12 months, providing them with information about their condition and the necessity for thyroid function testing.

Further reading

Wakley G, Chambers R and Pullan A (2004) *Demonstrating Your Competence 4: respiratory disease, mental health, diabetes and dermatology.* Radcliffe Publishing, Oxford.

References

1   Prodigy Guidelines on www.prodigy.nhs.uk/guidance.asp?gt=Hyperthyroidism

2   National Prescribing Centre (2001) Management of thyroid disease. *MeRec Bulletin.* **13(3)**: 9–12. www.npc.co.uk/MeReC_Bulletins/2001Volumes/pdfs/vol12no3.pdf

3 Danase MD, Ladenson PW, Meinert CL *et al.* (2000) Effect of thyroxine therapy on serum lipoproteins in patients with mild thyroid failure: a quantitative review of the literature. *Journal of Clinical Endocrinology and Metabolism.* **85**: 2993–3001.

4 Godlee F (ed.) (2004) *Clinical Evidence Concise. Issue 11.* BMJ Publishing Group, London. www.clinicalevidence.com

5 Vanderpump MP, Ahlquist JAO, Franklyn J *et al.* (1996) Consensus statement for good practice and audit measures in the management of hypothyroidism and hyperthyroidism. The Research Unit of the Royal College of Physicians, the Endocrinology and Diabetes Committee of the Royal College of Physicians and the Society for Endocrinology. *BMJ.* **313**: 539–44.

6 Joint Formulary Committee (2004) *British National Formulary. BNF 47.* British Medical Association and the Royal Pharmaceutical Society of Great Britain, London. www.bnf.org

8

Asthma

To explore how your primary care team might work together to improve the management of patients with asthma you can review a case (or cases) with which your team has been involved. You may prefer to use the two example cases at the start of this chapter. Read through them quickly before working on the problem case exercise (*see* page 113), or just photocopy Table 1.1 on page 7 to develop your own problem case. Include in your team people who will join in the problem-based learning discussion and be part of the solutions.

If you feel that you have insufficient knowledge to guide you in completing the problem-based learning, use the summary about asthma in the second part of this chapter and follow up the references if you need to learn more.

Example problem case 1

Problem Case:

An audit of the asthma register reveals that 53% of patients have no computer record of an asthma review in the past 15 months.

Who do you need in your team?

You might want a team that includes:

Reception staff
Practice manager
Practice nurses
District nurses
GPs
Patients and carers
IT staff.

Where you are now

Discussion between practice team members reveals:

- a member of the reception staff has been responsible for running the asthma clinic call and recall system on an *ad hoc* basis between her other reception duties.

- one of your practice nurses is responsible for carrying out asthma reviews. There are no protected appointment times for this, appointments being slotted in on a first come, first served basis. The nurse reports frequent non-attendance for asthma reviews
- the current waiting time for a practice nurse appointment is three weeks
- one of the doctors prefers to perform his own asthma reviews on his patients. He finds the practice computer asthma template difficult to use admitting that he seldom bothers using it, preferring to enter data as 'free text'
- a small number of asthma patients are housebound and do not receive a structured asthma review.

What you do next

This might include.

- A meeting between members of the primary care team to agree a common approach to performing and recording asthma reviews.
- Reviewing the role of the 'asthma clinic call and recall clerk'. Appropriate training given in protected time to adequately perform this task.
- Examining the availability of appointments with the practice nurse. The shortage of appointments prompts an audit of tasks performed. Analysis suggests that up to 40% of the work currently performed by the practice nurse could safely be delegated to a less qualified health professional. So you decide to employ an appropriately trained healthcare assistant.
- Contacting a sample of patients who missed their asthma review appointments to establish why. You find that 25% of patients had forgotten their appointment; 50% did not see the need for a review of their asthma; 5% were too ill to attend; and there was no response from 20%.
- Agreeing to emphasise the importance of regular reviews to asthma patients, opportunistically at patient contacts and by adding reminders to patients' prescriptions.
- Configuring the practice computer to indicate when a patient is more than one month overdue for review of their asthma.
- Examining the computer template used for asthma reviews. Arrange training in its use for all who need it. The doctor who previously expressed difficulties should now find the template easy to use.
- Entering the additional computer training received in your personal development plans.
- Reviewing the records of patients who have seen the doctor who has not used the asthma template and who are on salbutamol or terbutaline. Enter any asthma related data recovered in the appropriate areas of these patients' notes.
- Performing routine asthma reviews on housebound patients using a paper template to enter data. A GP reviews the completed paper template and the IT clerk subsequently enters the information onto the practice computer system.
- Completing Table 8.1.

What extra resources might this require?

- Time for initial meetings and for training.
- Protected time for the clerk administering the asthma call and recall system.

- Training in asthma management and administration of recall systems. IT training for those who are not confident using computerised templates.
- Educational resources for patients: availability of suitable leaflets and educational video material. Particular emphasis placed on the role and importance of regular follow-ups of asthma.
- Additional staffing hours will be needed, by modifying the workload of existing staff, extending the hours of existing staff or employing additional staff. A healthcare assistant may be the most cost-effective approach. If staff are used to improve asthma points score from the quality and outcomes framework, the additional costs may be covered by an increase in practice profits.
- The district nurse may seek help from practice employed staff to compensate for the extra work he or she is undertaking 'for the practice'.

The outcomes

These might include.

- a significant increase in the percentage of patients who have had an asthma review in the previous 15 months
- better uptake of asthma review appointments may produce increases in other asthma related quality markers such as smoking status, smoking advice and 'flu vaccination.

How would you demonstrate that you have achieved your outcomes?

Regular audits should show higher percentages of patients on the asthma register who:

- have had an asthma review in the past 15 months
- have smoking status recorded in the past 15 months
- smoke and have a record that smoking cessation advice has been given or referral offered within the past 15 months
- are aged 16 years or over who have asthma and have been given a 'flu vaccine in the preceding 1 September to 31 March.

Example problem case 2

Problem Case:

An audit of asthma medication ordered on repeat prescription by patients with asthma demonstrates that a cohort of patients is ordering insufficient inhaled steroids to provide the dosage prescribed. On discussing this result with a community pharmacist, she mentions anecdotal reports of patients ordering inhaled steroids 'to keep the doctor happy' but with no intention of using them.

Table 8.1: Role and responsibilities checklist – *for each task tick the box for each team member who has a role or responsibility – then note your role and responsibilities for the task*

Completed by: _____

Task	Primary care team member								What are your roles and your responsibilities?
	Doctor	*Practice nurse*	*District nurse*	*Reception team*	*Practice manager*	*Patients*	*IT clerk*	*Other*	
Identifying patients who should be included on the register	✔	✔	✔	✔	✔	✔	✔	✔	*e.g. Ensuring those with a confirmed diagnosis of asthma are on the register. Those where asthma has not been confirmed are reviewed and removed as indicated*
Ensuring asthma review call/recall system operates effectively		✔		✔	✔	✔	✔		*e.g. To ensure asthma patients are invited for regular review and to follow up those who do not attend*
Ensuring data is collected and entered appropriately in patient records	✔	✔	(✔)		✔		✔		*e.g. An appropriately trained district nurse may be involved in asthma reviews of housebound patients.* *Practice manager should oversee regular audits to check data is being collected and entered on the practice computer system*
Task 4									
Task 5									

Who do you need in your team?

You might want a team that includes:

Reception staff
Community pharmacist
Practice nurses
District nurses
GPs
Patients and carers
IT staff.

Where you are now

- A meeting is arranged between doctors, practice nurses, district nurses, the receptionist and the community pharmacist to discuss the audit findings. The interpretation placed on the audit results is that either:
  - patients who are not using their prescribed inhaled steroids no longer require these medications, *or*
  - although patients require the inhaled steroids prescribed they are not using them because they are unwilling to do so.
- On discussion at the meeting no one can recall stepping down asthma treatment for individual patients over the past six months. This impression is confirmed by an audit of repeat asthma prescriptions. The audit demonstrates no instances of reduced dose of inhaled steroids being prescribed. This suggests that some inhaled steroid prescriptions may not be clinically indicated.
- Further discussion reveals clinicians' unease at stepping down asthma treatments. Particular concerns raised are that it is difficult to know when to step down treatment and the risk of destabilising previously well controlled asthma.
- Various participants perceive that some patients remain unhappy about using inhaler steroids.

What you do next

This might include.

- Arranging a practice-based educational event with a consultant respiratory physician and an asthma nurse specialist as expert resources. Discussing best practice in the management of asthma. Emphasising when to step down asthma treatment and the exact procedures that should be followed.
- From this meeting, producing a set of guidelines detailing when and how to step down asthma treatment. Ensuring that the primary care team feel that they own the guidelines and follow local and national best practice.[1-5]
- Amending the asthma review computer template to include a prompt about stepping down treatment if appropriate.
- Sending a questionnaire concerning views on inhaled steroids to a sample group of asthma patients (or in the case of children, their carers). When you do, 30% of the responses indicate their anxiety regarding the use of inhaled steroids, the main concerns being 'risk of osteoporosis' in adult patients and 'growth retardation' in the case of children.

- Establishing a patient-centred education programme. This will include leaflets, video presentations in the waiting room and additional time during routine asthma reviews to allow for discussion.

What extra resources might this require?

- The practice-based educational meeting will require time to hold it and a suitable room in which to meet.
- Local experts may require remuneration in the form of speakers' fees.
- Time to produce the guidelines and costs of the paper on which to print or laminate them.
- Time to produce and to analyse a patient questionnaire and costs of printing, postage and secretarial time.
- Printed leaflets and additional medical and nursing time to provide sufficient information for concordance in asthma treatment for the patient education programme.

The outcomes

These might include.

- Medical and nursing staff who are confident about stepping down a patient's asthma treatment as indicated by agreed guidelines.
- Concordance reached with each patient as to their specific treatment regime.
- Asthma medication on prescription for any particular patient represents the medication actually being used by that patient.

How would you demonstrate that you have achieved your outcomes?

- An audit of prescription amendments for patients on the asthma register will identify some patients for whom treatment has been stepped down.
- An audit of repeat prescription use demonstrates that re-ordering of repeat prescriptions for regular preventive therapy (including inhaled steroids) accords with expected rate of use.
- A repeat survey of attitudes amongst asthma patients to inhaled steroids will establish if a change has occurred – at least in part due to the primary care team's educational efforts.

Problem case exercise

Problem Case:

A patient presents in surgery with acute severe asthma. The urgency of the problem is recognised. The patient is managed appropriately and after a two-day stay in hospital is discharged. This episode is used as the focus for a significant event analysis meeting.

The analysis, although generally favourable reveals two causes of concern.

1 The patient had requested and obtained a prescription for a salbutamol inhaler (four prescriptions in total) on four of the ten days before the episode of acute severe asthma.
2 The patient had no patient-held asthma management plan.

Who do you need in your team?

Where you are now

What you do next

Continued

What extra resources might this require?

The outcomes

How would you demonstrate that you have achieved your outcomes?

Why asthma is important

Eight million people in the UK have been diagnosed as having asthma. Just over five million are currently receiving treatment. On average 1400 people die from asthma each year in the UK. There were over 71 000 hospital admissions for asthma in the UK in 2001. An estimated 75% of hospital admissions for asthma are judged to be avoidable and as many as 90% of deaths from asthma preventable. Asthma costs the NHS £850 million a year and there is a loss of over 18 million working days.[1]

Importance of a proactive approach to asthma care

Routine clinical review of people with asthma is associated with favourable clinical outcomes including:

* reduced exacerbation rates
* improved symptom control
* reduced school or work absence rates.[2]

The following elements are required for proactive asthma care to be given.

* Diagnosis: to establish that patients are suffering from asthma.
* A register of patients with asthma is established and maintained.
* Routine reviews should follow appropriate guidelines and be undertaken by an appropriately trained doctor or nurse.
* Adjustment of a patient's treatment should be dictated by the degree of control of their asthma.
* A system to identify and contact those who default on their asthma review (although a patient has the right to decline an asthma review).
* A system to identify early signs of deteriorating asthma control, for example early ordering of reliever medication.
* Regular audit and practice systems adjusted according to audit outcomes.

The primary care team should be able to respond rapidly and appropriately to exacerbations of asthma.

Diagnosis of asthma in adults

Symptoms suggestive of asthma in adults are:

* wheeze
* shortness of breath
* chest tightness
* cough.

Symptoms may be variable and episodic. There may be no clinical signs. Alternatively the patient may have a diffuse, bilateral expiratory wheeze. An inspiratory wheeze may also be present. There may be a personal or family history of atopy, a history of worsening of symptoms after aspirin, non-steroidal anti-inflammatory drugs (NSAIDs) or beta-blockers or even a history of episodes of asthma being triggered by pollens, dust, animals, exercise, viral infections, chemicals or irritants.

Diagnosis should be confirmed by spirometry or by peak flow measurements in patients over the age of eight years old. Diagnosis may be made on *any* of the following criteria.[3]

* A greater than 20% diurnal variation on three or more days in a week for two weeks in a peak expiratory flow diary.
* Increase in FEV_1 by at least 15% (and 200 ml) after short acting beta-2-agonist given (e.g. salbutamol 400 mcg by pMDI + spacer or 2.5 mg via nebuliser).
* Increase in FEV_1 by at least 15% (and 200 ml) after trial of steroid tablets (prednisolone 30 mg/day for 14 days).
* Decrease in FEV_1 by at least 15% after six minutes of exercise (e.g. running).

Diagnosis of asthma in children

It can be difficult to reach a definitive diagnosis of asthma in young children. Presenting features include:

- wheeze
- dry cough
- breathlessness
- noisy breathing.

Asthma should be suspected in any child with wheezing ideally heard by a health professional on auscultation and distinguished from upper airways noise.[4] The diagnosis of asthma is reached by excluding other causes of presenting symptoms and by the child's favourable response to asthma treatment.

Asthma registers

All health professionals should take responsibility for ensuring newly diagnosed asthmatic patients are entered on the asthma register. It is usually kept on the practice's computer system so it is readily auditable and computer-generated invitations can be sent out to those on the register to attend the clinic. Set an alert attached to a patient's electronic medical record that will indicate if the patient is overdue for a routine asthma review. Responsibility for this usually lies with the audit or IT clerk.

Routine review of asthmatic patients[2]

The precise structure of an asthma clinic review varies according to local need. It may be run by a doctor, nurse or other appropriately trained healthcare professional. An example of the areas that may be addressed is shown in Box 8.1.

Box 8.1:　An asthma clinic review in general practice[6]

History
- Symptoms the patient is experiencing:
  - difficulty sleeping because of asthma symptoms
  - day-time symptoms (cough/wheeze/breathlessness/chest tightness)
  - interference with patient's usual activities
- What treatment(s) the patient is using:
  - how often reliever inhaler is required
- Any factors that trigger asthma attacks
- Smoking status
- Date of last asthma attack
- Whether patient has required hospitalisation
- Whether patient has required emergency steroids

Continued

Examination
- Check patient's peak flow
- Examine patient's peak flow diary
- Check patient's inhaler technique

Patient education
- Discuss smoking if relevant (consider referral to smoking cessation clinic)
- Discuss nature and avoidance of trigger factors
- Reinforce good inhaler technique
- Other appropriate health promotion areas, e.g. maintaining reasonable weight and taking regular exercise

Review or modify treatment (the degree of responsibility taken by a nurse depends on her training and capabilities)

- Review treatment: step up or down as appropriate
- If required, modify inhaler device used and teach patient technique for new inhaler device
- Review patient-held asthma management plan and modify if necessary (an example of a patient-held asthma management plan may be downloaded from the asthma UK website www.asthma.org.uk/pros/publications02.php).

The British Thoracic Society[6] and the Scottish Intercollegiate Guidelines Network[7,8] have produced a stepwise summary of the (pharmacological) management of asthma. These are reproduced in Boxes 8.2, 8.3 and 8.4.

Indicators of poorly controlled asthma may be indicated by:

- presence of symptoms
- frequent exacerbations
- high use of reliever medication.

These symptoms and signs should be seen as an indication to step up asthma treatment.

The patient's asthma and its treatment should be reviewed regularly. Where asthma is well controlled consider stepping down treatment, the aim being to maintain the patient at the lowest dose of inhaled steroid that controls the asthma. Reductions should be considered every three months, decreasing the dose by approximately 25 to 50% each time.[8]

Box 8.2:   Guidelines for the stepwise treatment of asthma in adults[5,8]

Treatment should be started at the step that seems most appropriate to the severity of the patient's asthma. The treatment may be stepped up or stepped down as dictated by the response and severity of the patient's asthma. The dose of inhaled steroid given refers to beclomethasone diproprionate or equivalent.

Step 1:   **Mild intermittent asthma**
Inhaled short acting beta-2-agonist as required

Step 2:   **Regular preventer therapy**
Add inhaled steroid 200–800 mcg/day

Step 3:   **Add-on therapy**
a   Add inhaled long-acting beta-2-agonist (LABA)
b   Assess control of asthma:
Good response to LABA – continue LABA
Benefits from LABA but control still inadequate – continue LABA and increase inhaled steroid dose to 800 mcg/day
No response to LABA – stop LABA and increase inhaled steroid to 800 mcg/day. If control still inadequate, institute trial of other therapies, e.g. leukotriene receptor antagonist, sustained release theophylline

Step 4:   **Persistent poor control**
Consider trials of:
Increasing inhaled steroid up to 2000 mcg/day
Addition of fourth drug, e.g. leukotriene receptor antagonist, sustained release theophylline, or oral beta-2-agonist

Step 5:   **Continuous or frequent use of oral steroids**
Use daily steroid dose in lowest dose providing adequate control
Maintain high-dose inhaled steroid at 2000 mcg/day
Consider other treatments to minimise steroid use
Refer patient to specialist care

Box 8.3: Guidelines for the stepwise treatment of asthma in children aged five to 12 years[5,8]

Treatment should be commenced at the step that seems most appropriate to the severity of the patient's asthma. The treatment may be stepped up or stepped down as dictated by the response and severity of the patient's asthma. The dose of inhaled steroid given refers to beclomethasone diproprionate or equivalent.

Step 1: **Mild intermittent asthma**
Inhaled short-acting beta-2-agonist as required

Step 2: **Regular preventer therapy**
Add inhaled steroid 200–400 mcg/day
Start at dose of inhaled steroid appropriate to severity of disease
200 mcg is an appropriate starting dose for many patients

Step 3: **Add-on therapy**
a Add inhaled long-acting beta-2-agonist (LABA)
b Assess control of asthma:
Good response to LABA – continue LABA
Benefits from LABA but control still inadequate – continue LABA and increase inhaled steroid dose to 400 mcg/day
No response to LABA – stop LABA and increase inhaled steroid to 400 mcg/day. If control still inadequate, institute trial of other therapies, e.g. leukotriene receptor antagonist, sustained release theophylline

Step 4: **Persistent poor control**
Increasing inhaled steroid up to 800 mcg/day

Step 5: **Continuous or frequent use of oral steroids**
Use daily steroid dose in lowest dose providing adequate control
Maintain high-dose inhaled steroid at 800 mcg/day
Refer patient to respiratory paediatrician

Box 8.4:   Guidelines for stepwise treatment of asthma in children less than five years old [5,8]

Treatment should be started at the step that seems most appropriate to the severity of the patient's asthma. The treatment may be stepped up or stepped down as dictated by the response and severity of the patient's asthma. The dose of inhaled steroid given refers to beclomethasone diproprionate or equivalent.

Step 1:   **Mild intermittent asthma**
           Inhaled short-acting beta-2-agonist as required

Step 2:   **Regular preventer therapy**
           Add inhaled steroid 200–400 mcg/day
           Or leukotriene receptor agonist if inhaled steroid cannot be used
           Start at dose of inhaled steroid appropriate to severity of disease

Step 3:   **Add-on therapy**
           In children aged two to five years consider trial of leukotriene receptor agonist
           If child under two years consider proceeding to *Step 4*

Step 4:   **Persistent poor control**
           Refer patient to respiratory paediatrician

Outcomes

Outcomes that indicate good asthma care include the following.

- Patients having no or few current symptoms.
- Patients able to use prescribed inhalers effectively.
- Patients with normal lung function ($FEV_1 > 85\%$).
- Patients with actual PEFR > 85% normal or best.
- Patients with an asthma management plan.

The GMS contract recognises the importance of asthma by attaching a points value to certain easily measurable quality indicators as detailed in Table 8.2.

Table 8.2: Quality and outcomes measures for asthma[9]

Criteria	Maximum thresholds (minimum 25%) (%)	Points
Register of patients with asthma (excluding those who have not been prescribed asthma related drugs in last 12 months)	Consistent with local Prevalence	7
Percentage of patients aged eight years and over who have been diagnosed as having asthma from 1 April 2003 have had the diagnosis confirmed by spirometry or peak flow measurement	70	15
Percentage of patients with asthma between the ages of 14 and 19 years who have a record of smoking status in the previous 15 months	70	6
Percentage of patients aged 20 years and over with asthma who have a record of smoking status in the past 15 months, except those who have never smoked where smoking status has been recorded at least once	70	6
Percentage of patients with asthma who smoke who have a record that smoking cessation advice or referral to a specialist service, if available, has been offered within the last 15 months	70	6
Percentage of patients with asthma who have had an asthma review in the last 15 months	70	20
Percentage of patients aged 16 years and over with asthma who have had 'flu immunisation in the preceding 1 September to 31 March	70	12

Asthma resources

Asthma UK
www.asthma.org.uk/index.php Home page.
www.asthma.org.uk/pros/resources.php Resources for health professionals.

British Thoracic Society
www.brit-thoracic.org.uk/ Home page
www.brit-thoracic.org.uk/sign/index.htm Site for download of BTS/SIGN guidelines

Clinical Evidence
www.clinicalevidence.com/ceweb/conditions/index.jsp

General Practice Airways Group
www.gpiag.org/

National Institute for Clinical Excellence
www.nice.org.uk/page.aspx?o=home

References

1   Asthma UK website: key facts and statistics. www.asthma.org.uk/journalists/facts.php#1

2   British Thoracic Society/Scottish Intercollegiate Guidelines Network (2003) British Guidelines on the Management of Asthma. *Thorax.* **58(Suppl 1)**: i54.

3   British Thoracic Society/Scottish Intercollegiate Guidelines Network (2003) British Guidelines on the Management of Asthma. *Thorax.* **58(Suppl 1)**: i5.

4   British Thoracic Society/Scottish Intercollegiate Guidelines Network (2003) British Guidelines on the Management of Asthma. *Thorax.* **58(Suppl 1)**: i6.

5   Chambers R, Wakley G and Pullan A (2005) *Demonstrating Your Competence 4: respiratory disease, mental health, diabetes and dermatology.* Radcliffe Publishing, Oxford.

6   The British Thoracic Society, 17 Doughty Street, London EC1N 2PL. www.brit-thoracic.org.uk

7   Scottish Intercollegiate Guidelines Network (SIGN), Royal College of Physicians, 9 Queen Street, Edinburgh EH2 1JQ. www.sign.ac.uk

8   British Thoracic Society/Scottish Intercollegiate Guidelines Network (2003) British Guidelines on the Management of Asthma. *Thorax.* **58(Suppl 1)**: i27.

9   General Practitioners Committee/The NHS Confederation (2003) *New GMS Contract 2003. Investing in General Practice.* British Medical Association, London.

9

Mental health

To explore how your primary care team might work together to improve the management of patients with mental health problems you can review a case (or cases) with which your team has been involved. You may prefer to use the two example cases at the start of this chapter. Read through them quickly before working on the problem case exercise (*see* page 128), or just photocopy Table 1.1 on page 7 to develop your own problem case. Include in your team people who will join in the problem-based learning discussion and be part of the solutions.

If you feel that you have insufficient knowledge to guide you in completing the problem-based learning, use the summary about mental health problems in the second part of this chapter and follow up the references if you need to learn more.

Example problem case 1

Problem Case:

Although the practice team think that they have managed to identify most of those with severe continuing mental health problems, obtaining consent for recording those patients on a register for recall and review has been more difficult. They had been surprised to find out from the PCO that they needed to obtain consent from individual patients before sending them for review.

Who do you want in your team?

You might want a team that includes:

Reception staff
Practice manager
Practice nurses
District nurses
GPs
Patients and carers
Pharmacists
Residential home staff
Community psychiatric nurses (CPNs).

Where you are now

The practice team had consulted the BMA website and had decided to ask for written consent for patients to be recorded.[1] The quality and outcomes framework for mental health level 1 states that: 'The practice can produce a register of people with severe long-term mental health problems who require and *have agreed to regular follow-up*'. The advice from the BMA was that patients have to be asked and they have to agree. Implied consent is not sufficient.

Letters with a consent form had been sent out to those identified. Several of the patients listed had not been seen by anyone in the practice for some time. Despite the stamped addressed envelope for the return of the consent form, hardly any were sent back.

What you do next

This might include.

- Consulting the information available from the National Primary Care Research and Development Centre (NPCRDC)[2] about how to implement the National Service Framework (NSF) for Mental Health[3] and satisfy the requirements of the quality and outcomes framework.
- Reviewing the letter sent out to patients with mental health problems. Obtain the views of community psychiatric nurses (CPNs), some of the patients on the list of patients with long-term disabling mental health problems who attend the surgery, carers and key workers. You might ask a local charity such as MIND or Age Concern for its advice. Modify the information sent out to make the advantages of regular contact more attractive and obvious.
- Obtaining consent personally when people listed for the register are in contact with a health professional at the surgery. Ask for help from the CPN, key workers and carers. You might use the re-designed letter as an information resource. Include this when patients are asked to attend for medication review and offer health checks at the same time.
- Providing more information about resources and help available to people with mental health problems around the practice premises and advertising this to patients. Arrange for leaflets, posters and contact details about voluntary societies or an information computer screen from the library service to be on display in the waiting room or on the wall of a corridor. Many practices offer sessions run by a Citizens' Advice Bureau in return for a rent-free room.
- Completing Table 9.1.

What extra resources might this require?

- The practice designated lead on mental health will need time to read the information from the NPCRDC, review the letter and rewrite it.[2] He/she may require secretarial time.
- Postage costs will have to be repeated to contact all of those who have not responded.
- A meeting at which the practice lead on mental health informs all the practice team about the register and its advantages, so that everyone that patients encounter knows about it and can explain it.
- The practice lead will need time to contact the CPNs, key workers and any carers who have queries about the new arrangements.

- Schedule longer appointments for the medication review of people with mental health problems so that screening tests can be offered and explained, and the advantages of regular review explained. Give the revised information letter to patients to take away with them, if they want more time to consider it.
- The practice lead can delegate the collection of suitable resources that will benefit patients as above, but the person involved will need time and expertise to do this – this might fall to the practice manager if negotiations are required about access to the practice premises.

The outcomes

- Informed consent from the majority of patients with concordance, not compliance, for health interventions. (See page 172 if you are not clear about the difference.)
- Improved co-operation between the primary care team, CPNs, key workers and carers of people with long-term and disabling mental health problems.
- Improved understanding by all of the primary healthcare team of the difficulties that this group of patients have in accessing health care.
- Improved information about resources and services that will benefit all patients.

How would you demonstrate that you have achieved your outcomes?

- A high proportion of patients listed as having long-term and disabling mental health problems give informed consent to being on the register for regular review.
- Information resources in the practice are more obviously available.
- The practice lead for mental health has a list of known people who care for patients listed with long-term and disabling mental health problems.

Example problem case 2

> **Problem Case:**
>
> A search of the records of patients receiving lithium prescriptions finds low levels of recording of lithium levels and little evidence of thyroid function and creatinine tests having been done.

Who do you need in your team?

You might want a team that includes:

Patients and carers
Practice nurses
GPs
Clerical staff
Pharmacists
Practice manager

Table 9.1: Role and responsibilities checklist – *for each task tick the box for each team member who has a role or responsibility – then note your role and responsibilities for the task*

Completed by: _____

Task	Primary care team member							What are your roles and your responsibilities?
	Doctor	*Practice nurse*	*District nurse*	*CPN*	*Practice manager*	*Patients*	*Other*	
Identifying patients who should be included on the register	✔	✔	✔	✔	✔	✔	✔	*e.g. Making sure that people who have not given consent are **not** included on the register*
Task 2								
Task 3								
Task 4								
Task 5								

CPNs and key workers
Day hospital staff.

Where you are now

Local arrangements for lithium monitoring were taken over by the day centre when it was established. Patients attend on a designated day and time for monitoring and are advised directly if they need to change their dose. This results in patients or pharmacists altering repeat medication requests and staff responsible for repeat prescriptions have got into the habit of ringing the day centre to confirm what dose people are taking, rather than bothering the doctor. Copies of the results of lithium levels or other blood tests have not been sent routinely to the practice, but the system appears to be working well otherwise.

What you do next

This might include.

- Talking to the staff at the day centre about how to resolve the problem, perhaps by asking them to write blood test results and any medication change on the repeat prescription, or in a co-operation booklet like that used for anticoagulant monitoring, held by the patient.
- Trying to involve the patients and their carers in taking responsibility for promptly passing on blood test results and any changes in medication to the practice.
- Entering the results of blood tests and medication changes into the electronic medical record.
- A fail-safe system to pick up anyone continuing to request medication without attending the day centre for monitoring.
- Liaising with the relevant pharmacies to explain the new system.

What extra resources might this require?

- Time for the responsible person at the practice to talk to the day centre staff, pharmacists and patients concerned.
- Time for a receptionist/secretary to enter blood results into the electronic medical record so that information can be readily retrieved.
- Time for the prescriber to check that blood results have been recorded before renewing time-limited repeat prescriptions.

The outcomes

These might include.

- Improved and retrievable recording of monitoring blood tests for people taking lithium.
- A fail-safe mechanism to ensure people do not continue to take lithium without monitoring.

How would you demonstrate that you have achieved your outcomes?

- A search shows that you easily achieve the standard of 90% of patients on lithium having had their blood tests within the recommended times.

- An audit shows that repeat prescriptions for lithium are not renewed without evidence of a lithium blood level in the last six months, or tests for thyroid function and creatinine having been done in the last 12 months.

Problem case exercise

Problem Case:

The implementation lead for the Mental Health NSF in the PCO has written to practices asking for copies of their protocols for managing mental health problems such as depression, postnatal depression, substance abuse, etc.[3] He writes that he expects these to be up to date and in line with current recommendations.

Who do you need in your team?

Where you are now

What you do next

Continued

What extra resources might this require?

The outcomes

How would you demonstrate that you have achieved your outcomes?

Why mental health is important

At any one time, one adult in six suffers from one or other form of mental illness. It is about as common as asthma. Mental health problems range from common conditions such as anxiety or depression, to psychotic illnesses such as schizophrenia or bipolar affective disorder (manic depression) that only affect one person in 250.[3]

The primary healthcare team looks after most people with mental health problems. However, some people with severe and enduring mental illness need care from specialist services working in partnership with the independent sector and agencies that provide housing, training and employment. Specialist services, including social care, should ensure effective and timely interventions for individuals whose mental health problems cannot be managed in primary care alone; for example, those patients with severe depression or psychotic disorders. Specialist services are essential when these problems exist together with substance misuse. Working partnerships with agencies that provide housing, training, help with finance or employment and leisure services are required to meet the needs of some people with enduring mental health needs. Standards two and three of the *NSF*[3] apply to services in primary care.

Standard two

Any service user who contacts their primary healthcare team with a common mental health problem should:

- have their mental health needs identified and assessed
- be offered effective treatments, including referral to specialist services for further assessment, treatment and care if they require it.

Standard three

Any individual with a common mental health problem should:

- be able to make contact round the clock with local services necessary to meet their needs and receive adequate care
- be able to use *NHS Direct* for first-level advice and referral on to specialist helplines or to local services.

People with mental health problems also suffer from poor physical health and are more prone to life-threatening illnesses due to poor diet, lifestyle and long-term effects of psychiatric medication. Worldwide, mental illness accounts for about 1.4% of all deaths and more than a quarter of the years lived with disability. In 1990, five of the ten leading causes of disability were psychiatric conditions: unipolar depression, alcohol misuse, bipolar affective disorder, schizophrenia and obsessive-compulsive disorder. People with severe mental illness are also socially excluded, finding it difficult to sustain social and family networks, access education systems and obtain and sustain employment. In a pooled analysis of 20 studies of 36 000 people, mortality among people with schizophrenia was found to be 1.6 times that of the general population; the risk of suicide was nine times higher; and the risk of death from other violent incidents over twice as high.[3]

Depression

Each year, one woman in every 15 and one man in every 30 will be affected by depression, and every GP will see between 60 and 100 people with depression.[3] Most of the 4000 suicides committed each year in England are attributed to depression. A review of the literature concluded that depression can be a major risk factor in cardiovascular and cerebrovascular disease and for death after a myocardial infarction.[3] Depression can also be associated with chronic physical illness such as arthritis, stroke or heart disease.

Depression can affect other family members. The emotional and cognitive development of socially deprived children of a depressed mother is especially affected, with boys more vulnerable than girls. Depression in people from the African-Caribbean, Asian, refugee and asylum seeker communities in the UK is frequently overlooked.[3]

From compliance to concordance

Research has shown that around 8% of prescriptions for antidepressants are never dispensed.[4] Many drugs that are dispensed are not consumed. At least 25 to 50% of patients on antidepressant medication take irregular or insufficient doses. You should find ways to encourage patients to adhere to the drugs prescribed for them. Give them better information so that they can take part in the decision to take antidepressants and be more likely to 'own' that agreement.[5]

Severe and long-term mental illness

'Severe and enduring mental illness' is covered by standards four and five of the NSF.[3] At present people with these conditions are likely to be those covered by the quality and outcomes framework.

Standard four

All mental health service users on the Care Programme Approach (CPA) should:

- receive care which optimises engagement, prevents or anticipates crisis, and reduces risk
- have a copy of a written care plan which:
  - includes action to be taken in a crisis by service users, their carers, and their care co-ordinators
  - advises the GP how they should respond if the service user needs additional help
  - is regularly reviewed by the care co-ordinator
- be able to access services 24 hours a day, 365 days a year.

Standard five

Each service user who is assessed as requiring a period of care away from their home should have:

- timely access to an appropriate hospital bed or alternative bed or place, which is:
  - in the least restrictive environment consistent with the need to protect them and the public
  - as close to home as possible

- a copy of a written after-care plan agreed on discharge, which sets out the care and rehabilitation to be provided, identifies the care co-ordinator and specifies the action to be taken in a crisis.

What mental health problems are included in the NSF?

People with 'severe long-term mental health problems' are described in the *NSF for Mental Health*[3] as 'patients who are managed by the care plan approach'. These may include patients:

- suffering from severe or recurrent depression
- suffering from bipolar depression
- with a history of psychosis
- with drug and/or alcohol addiction.

It is not explicit whether all PCOs will include severe and enduring depression within the umbrella of 'severe long-term mental health problems' or will assume the term mainly applies to psychotic illnesses. You may want to consider some of the points from the *NSF* for further action in your practice or PCO. For example, you could consider the area covered by standard seven – preventing suicide – as your priority area for action in the mental health domain after you have covered the essential areas in the quality and outcomes framework.

Standard seven

Local health and social care communities should prevent suicides by:

- promoting mental health for all, working with individuals and communities
- delivering high-quality primary mental health care
- ensuring that anyone with a mental health problem can contact local services via the primary care team, a helpline or an A&E department
- ensuring that individuals with severe and enduring mental illness have a care plan which meets their specific needs, including access to services round the clock
- providing safe hospital accommodation for individuals who need it
- enabling individuals caring for someone with severe mental illness to receive the support which they need to continue to care.

And in addition:

- supporting local prison staff in preventing suicides among prisoners
- ensuring that staff are competent to assess the risk of suicide among individuals at greatest risk
- developing local systems for suicide audit to learn lessons and take any necessary action.

What should you do, when and how?

Setting up the register

- Define who your register should include with the agreement of the lead implementation officer in your PCO.
- Identify this group of patients by running a search and/or trawling medical records for diagnoses of psychotic illness and patients with a care programme.
- Search for patients who are receiving repeat medication for antipsychotics (oral and depot), anticholinergics, antidepressants and anxiolytics. Review the medical records to determine which of these patients falls into the defined group with long-term mental health problems and add them to the list.
- Compare your list with that of the community health team.
- Decide how to obtain informed consent from patients on this list. You might want to do this by letter initially, explaining the purpose of the register and benefits for those registered, asking people to return a consent form. You will probably need to follow this up by discussion with individual patients.
- Record the patients who have given consent on the mental health register.

Setting up annual reviews

- Identify who will be responsible for the call and recall of patients on the mental health register.
- Decide who will carry out reviews and if the practice staff involved require any further training. Reviews should include:
  - preventive care such as blood pressure, cervical screening
  - health education advice about smoking, diet and exercise
  - issues around alcohol or illegal drug use
  - medication review (if not being done elsewhere)
  - the risk of diabetes from atypical antipsychotics, e.g. risperidone and olanzapine
  - checking the co-ordination arrangements with others caring for the patients, including contact details and services required.

Lithium medication

- Search for patients who have received prescriptions for lithium in the preceding year.
- Audit the numbers who have results of their lithium levels, thyroid function and creatinine tests in their records. If results are missing, establish if they can be obtained from other sources, such as hospital letters.
- Make an action plan for improving the level of recording. You may need to:
  - limit the issues of repeat prescriptions for lithium to establish a system to pick up any overdue tests and issue reminders
  - ensure that results from tests carried out elsewhere, e.g. in a 'lithium clinic' or day centre, are recorded in the medical records
  - agree a protocol to clarify who is responsible for monitoring – primary care or secondary care
  - the therapeutic range for lithium is usually 0.6–1.0 mmol/l. If the range acceptable locally is different, you will need to inform the PCO. Levels below this therapeutic range are acceptable for some individuals, depending on the clinical condition.

What are the outcomes?

These will include the quality and outcome indicators in mental health as in Table 9.2.

Table 9.2: Quality and outcomes measures for mental health

Criteria	Maximum thresholds (minimum 25%) (%)	Points
The practice can produce a register of patients who require, and have agreed to, regular follow-up	Practice is able to justify why patients have been included	7
A review is recorded in the last 15 months. The review includes a check on medication, physical health and co-ordination with secondary care	90	23
Patients on lithium have a record that the lithium level has been checked in the last six months	90	3
Patients on lithium have a record of their serum creatinine and thyroid function in the last 15 months	90	3
Patients on lithium have a record that the lithium level has been in the therapeutic range in the last six months	70	5

The guidance for the quality and outcomes framework accepts that it is impossible to define which patients should be included in the mental health register. The guidance suggests including patients who:

• have a psychotic illness
• are being treated under a care programme approach
• require a complex care package from a multidisciplinary secondary care team.

Much of the information for collating the register will come from secondary care. Set up procedures to record this information in the electronic medical record so that tests are not repeated unnecessarily and uneconomically.

These indicators are only a fraction of the work necessary to care for people with mental health problems and the burden of anxiety and depression is much larger. You may want to plan for developments in measuring outcomes for patients with *these* conditions, especially those with long-term problems.

What are the challenges?

A review of mental health services found shortages of skilled staff, problems in recruiting experienced managers and years of under-investment in information systems.[6] Staff and service users often worked in unacceptable environments.

Lack of co-operation and communication between the different sectors of social services, mental health teams, primary care, housing, etc. make care fragmented and often of an unacceptable standard. People with severe mental health problems are not able to demand better standards of care while they are ill, and their carers too are often desperate and worn down with the battle of trying to obtain care.

People with mental health problems often ignore their general health, or their mental health makes care for other problems more difficult. More time may be required to explain the purpose of screening or investigations to someone who has paranoid suspicions, a poor attention span or poor comprehension. Many patients who commit suicide have had recent contact with primary care, but not necessarily about mental health problems.

People with mental health problems, particularly those with co-existent drug and alcohol problems may find it difficult to register with a GP.

What can you do to make it more likely that you will succeed?

- Ensure that you record the contact details for anyone involved in caring for someone with mental health problems, e.g. a key worker or CPN so that the primary care team knows whom to contact when there are problems.
- Arrange for people with mental health problems to have screening tests, e.g. blood pressure checks, cervical screening. See that tests are adequately explained.
- Inform the PCO of examples of deficiencies of care.
- Play your part in the communication of information between providers – mental health teams equally complain that changes in medication or health are not passed on to them from primary care.
- Make sure that you understand clearly what is meant by 'obtaining consent'. The BMA produces a useful toolkit that can be downloaded from their website.[7]
- Ensure that your practice is accessible to those with severe mental health problems, e.g. those with drug or alcohol problems as well as psychotic illnesses.
- Provide training so that primary care staff have the requisite attitudes, skills and knowledge to deal effectively with mental health problems.
- The primary care team needs training to identify those at risk of suicide or self-harm.

Further reading

Chambers R, Wakley G and Pullan A (2004) *Demonstrating Your Competence 4: respiratory disease, mental health, diabetes and dermatology.* Radcliffe Publishing, Oxford.

References

1 Advice on consent for recording patients on the mental health register. www.bma.org.uk/ap.nsf/Content/faqschap30304?OpenDocument&Highlight=2,mental,health,consent

2 www.npcrdc.man.ac.uk/Publications/mentalhealth-handbook.pdf

3   National Health Service Executive (2000) *National Service Framework for Mental Health.* Department of Health, London. Full version: www.dh.gov.uk/assetRoot/04/07/72/09/04077209.pdf and executive summary on: www.dh.gov.uk/assetRoot/04/01/45/01/04014501.pdf

4   Johnston D (1981) Depression: treatment compliance in general practice. *Acta Psychiatrica Scandinavica.* **63(Suppl)**: 447–53.

5   Marinker M (ed.) (1997) *From Compliance to Concordance: achieving shared goals in medicine taking.* Royal Pharmaceutical Society; Merck, Sharp and Dohme, London.

6   Commission for Health Improvement report on Mental Health Trusts between 2001–2003: www.chi.nhs.uk/eng/cgr/mentalhealth/mentalhealthreport03.pdf

7   British Medical Association Consent Toolkit: www.bma.org.uk/ap.nsf/Content/consenttk2/$file/toolkit.pdf

10

Coronary heart disease

To explore how your primary care team might work together to improve the management of patients with coronary heart disease you can review a case (or cases) with which your team has been involved. You may prefer to use the two example cases at the start of this chapter. Read through them quickly before working on the problem case exercise (*see* page 142), or just photocopy Table 1.1 on page 7 to develop your own problem case. Include in your team people who will join in the problem-based learning discussion and be part of the solutions.

If you feel that you have insufficient knowledge to guide you in completing the problem-based learning, use the summary about coronary heart and cardiovascular disease in the second part of this chapter and follow up the references if you need to learn more.

Example problem case 1

> **Problem Case:**
>
> A clinical audit finds that 90% of patients on the coronary heart disease (CHD) register have aspirin, and over 70% have beta-blocker and ACE inhibitor drugs listed on their repeat prescription medication. However, the audit also shows that fewer than half of these patients are requesting medication regularly enough to cover their needs over a 12-month period.

Who do you need in your team?

You might want a team that includes:

Patient or carer and/or pharmacist or nursing home staff requesting regular repeat medication
Reception staff doing repeat prescriptions or recalling patients
Practice manager
Nurses and doctors seeing patients for other conditions
Secondary care staff initiating medication.

Where you are now

Looking at the clinical audit figures more closely you see that because patients have not requested their medication, a recall for review has not been triggered. You have no system for recording aspirin medication purchased by the patient over the counter (OTC).

What you do next

This might include.

- Establishing whether the medication repeats are being recorded accurately. Health professionals may be writing prescriptions by hand that are not captured by the system. For example, you may find that prescriptions for home visits are handwritten and not recorded as repeat prescriptions, or that one or two doctors handwrite prescriptions if the patient is consulting in person and asks for repeat medication.
- Setting up a method of recording reported OTC aspirin use by patients at each review appointment.
- Obtaining the views of patients on medication and their reasons why they do not request medication regularly.
- Looking at the literature in the library about why people do not take medication.
- Looking at the patient information leaflets given to patients after they have had a diagnosis of coronary heart disease made and seeing if you think it is good enough.
- Asking for feedback from patients about the information that they have received from doctors and nurses they have consulted.
- Using real or fictional case scenarios about patients taking their medication (or not) in an amusing way at an educational session so that staff can understand the need for concordance. Rehearse explaining the reasons for the treatment of coronary heart disease with each case.
- Carrying out regular clinical audit to find people on the register who have not been reviewed and inviting them for a health check (and review of their medication).
- Completing Table 10.1.

What extra resources might this require?

- Increased motivation of prescribers to use the computerised repeat prescription system by linking to the rewards received from the quality and outcomes framework.
- Training for those prescribers who are unfamiliar with the system of recording and issuing computerised prescriptions.
- Time and expertise to set up a short template for recording the medication review that captures OTC use of aspirin and contraindications to, or refusal of, medications.
- Time to train all health professionals in the use of the template.
- Staff time and skills for obtaining feedback from patients on the quality and completeness of the information they have received about their condition.
- Time to look at the literature in the library about medication compliance and the information patients receive about management of coronary heart disease.
- Time and resources for a staff educational session.
- Clerical time for doing the clinical audit data collection.

The outcomes

These might include.

- Repeat audits showing that the repeat prescribing system records an increasing number of patients as having regular repeats of their medication.
- OTC aspirin use is recorded consistently.
- Contraindications to, and refusals of, medication are recorded consistently.

How would you demonstrate that you have achieved your outcomes?

Repeat clinical audit at intervals to measure progress towards the targets.
   (For a problem case example of left ventricular dysfunction see Chapter 4, page 60.)

Example problem case 2

Problem Case:

The clerk responsible for maintaining the CHD register for the practice and auditing the quality and outcomes criteria complains to the practice manager that she enters the smoking status when it is known but no one else appears to be doing so when patients consult. She has also found that no record of smoking cessation advice is being recorded. She feels that this will reflect badly on her efforts to provide accurate information for the quality and outcomes framework.

Who do you need in your team?

You might want a team that includes:

Reception staff
Practice manager
Clerical and secretarial staff
Practice nurses
Midwives
District nurses
Health visitors
Doctors.

Where you are now

- Recording of patients' smoking status is not being done in a systematic way. The only time people are asked consistently is when the practice nurse sees them when they register as new patients.
- The doctors and nurses say they have insufficient time to ask people about their smoking habits. Other clinical matters take priority and they do not think about it.
- Entering information about smoking history on to the computer requires too much effort.

Table 10.1: Role and responsibilities checklist – *for each task tick the box for each team member who has a role or responsibility – then note your role and responsibilities for the task*

Completed by: _____

Task	Primary care team member							What are your roles and your responsibilities?
	Doctor	*Practice nurse*	*Patients*	*Reception team*	*Practice manager*	*Pharmacist*	*Other*	
Identifying patients who should be included on the register	✔	✔	✔	✔	✔	✔	✔	*e.g. Making sure that people suspected but not confirmed, of having the condition are **not** included on the register*
Task 2								
Task 3								
Task 4								
Task 5								

- Although the doctors and nurses say they are advising people about smoking cessation, no information about this is recorded anywhere.

What you do next

This might include.

- The reception staff handing out forms to patients to complete when they are attending the doctors, nurses, district nurses, health visitors and midwives.
- Attaching forms to repeat prescriptions for a four- to six-week period.
- All staff seeing patients, including district nurses, health visitors and midwives, agreeing to reinforce the information about why patients should complete the form. Those visiting patients at home take some forms with them for patients to complete.
- The form asks patients to complete their name, current address and telephone number(s) and lifestyle information about smoking. Corrections can then be made to addresses and telephone numbers.
- The form also asks if patients are interested in smoking cessation for themselves and directs them to collect information from the reception desk when handing over the form or placing in collection box, prominently displayed. The receptionist stamps the form to state that smoking cessation advice has been given.
- Boxes of cards and leaflets about the smoking cessation service being prominently displayed at the reception desk and there are posters around the reception area.
- The form also being used to advise patients that they should have their blood pressure checked if it has not been done in the last year and suggesting that they can book with the practice nurse to have this done.
- Once most of the information about smoking is computerised, an alerting flag will be set up on the computer for patients who have no information recorded, or who smoke but have not had their smoking history updated in the last 12 months. The nurses and doctors will have a relatively small number of people to ask and will not feel so overwhelmed that they cannot occasionally include this in consultations about other matters.

What extra resources might this require?

- The form has to be designed, piloted and printed.
- Reception staff need extra time to hand the form out, time to explain it to patients and receive the forms back, stamping them if necessary.
- Set aside dedicated time for clerical staff to enter information from the forms.
- Allow extra appointment time for the practice nurse to be available to take blood pressures, or train staff to do this.
- Expertise to set up an alerting flag on the computer for smoking history to be updated, linked to an entry about smoking cessation advice.
- Training for nurses and doctors to respond appropriately to the alerting flag.
- The clerk responsible will need time to carry out repeat audits to monitor progress.
- The practice manager needs time and skills to motivate the team and feedback on progress.

The outcomes

These might include.

- An increased percentage of patients have their smoking status recorded over the period of a year.
- An increased percentage of smokers are recorded as having received smoking cessation advice.
- Repeat auditing shows that the proportion of patients who have their smoking history and smoking cessation advice recorded is increasing each quarter benefiting not just this clinical domain but overlapping domains.
- An increased number of smokers who have pledged to quit receive nicotine replacement therapy.

How would you demonstrate that you have achieved your outcomes?

Regular repeat clinical audits.

Problem case exercise

Problem Case:

Two patients referred to the rapid access chest pain clinic re-attend with further episodes of pain. They both say that they have not received an appointment. You instigate a significant event audit and find that several people in the practice team were unaware that the arrangements made by the clinic were to fax appointments to the surgery rather than notifying the patients directly.

Who do you need in your team?

Where you are now

Continued

What you do next

What extra resources might this require?

The outcomes

How would you demonstrate that you have achieved your outcomes?

Why coronary heart disease and cardiovascular disease are important

Cardiovascular disease is a major cause of premature death in most European and North American populations. Myocardial infarction, stroke and death may occur suddenly in situations remote from medical care. Modification of risk factors has been shown to reduce mortality and morbidity.[1]

What is it?

The underlying cause of death is thought to be arteriosclerosis, which develops gradually over many years without symptoms until the condition is advanced. The current strategy for medical intervention is to focus on those who are at highest risk of coronary heart disease.

1   Primary prevention for individuals at high absolute risk of developing arteriosclerosis.
2   Secondary prevention for those with established cardiovascular disease.

More general population approaches such as reducing smoking by the government passing new laws, promoting healthy eating, increasing exercise and reducing obesity, are likely to have greater effects on long-term risk levels in the whole population. Health professionals can influence the initiatives made by governmental and non-governmental bodies, but cannot be wholly responsible for their implementation.

Assessment of risk

Absolute risk is the probability of developing coronary heart disease over a defined period. It can be established using *risk prediction charts*, of which there are a bewildering number. Most clinical computer systems have a chart available for use, or one can be downloaded from the web. The Joint British Societies Coronary Risk Prediction Chart is available in the *British National Formulary*[2] or *Guidelines*.[3]

Risk factors for coronary heart disease include:

- hypertension
- smoking
- high levels of total and low-density lipoproteins (LDLs)
- low levels of high-density lipoproteins (HDLs)
- diabetes
- increasing age in males of all ages and postmenopausal females
- family history of cardiovascular disease at an early age
- obesity (waist to hip ratio)
- some ethnic groups have increased risks.

Established coronary heart disease, stroke or peripheral vascular disease make someone a high risk automatically and a candidate for secondary preventive measures. Risk factors may be multi-factorial, or someone may have a very high level of one risk factor. An individual with diabetes or familial hypercholesteraemia would have a high risk even without any other risk factors.

What should you do, when and how?

Primary prevention

BEHAVIOURAL CHANGE

It is difficult, but not impossible, to help people make significant changes in their health behaviour. It is harder for people to change if they are socially disadvantaged or have low income, are unemployed or in jobs with little control of their situation, and under stress at work or home. Targeting lifestyle changes to prevent cardiovascular disease requires that someone is interested in changing, progresses to preparation to change, and then to making changes. People may relapse after making changes and need encouragement to repeat the process and maintain the changes made.

SMOKING

There is no safe level of smoking. All patients should be advised to stop and you can refer them to a smoking cessation service in your practice or a local community resource.

HEALTHY EATING

A good diet can modify several risk factors. It can reduce excess weight and blood pressure, control blood glucose levels, alter the ratio between high- and low-density lipoproteins and reduce triglyceride levels, and decrease the likelihood of thrombosis.

PHYSICAL ACTIVITY

Advise all patients without contraindications to take at least 20 to 30 minutes of vigorous exercise most days of the week, building up to this if they are inactive. More moderate exercise is still of benefit, if this cannot be achieved because of other health problems. Moderate to high activity significantly reduces the likelihood of coronary heart disease and stroke.[4]

REDUCTION OF RISKS FROM OTHER CONDITIONS

Good control of diabetes is essential to the reduction of risk from CHD.

MEDICATION

Consider treatment with statins for those people with a 30% or more ten-year absolute risk of coronary heart disease, that is there is at least a three in ten chance that they will have a major coronary event in the ensuing ten years.[2] People at lower risk may want advice about purchasing simvastatin from pharmacies. The amount of benefit is related to an individual's baseline risk and degree of cholesterol lowering, rather than the person's cholesterol concentration.[4] The *National Service Framework for Coronary Heart Disease*[5] advises that you use the Joint British Heart Society Charts.[2,3] Use the ratio of total cholesterol to high-density lipoprotein (HDL) to interpret the risk charts. Medication is mainly used for those needing secondary prevention. Anybody with diabetes is regarded as high risk and should take a statin, whatever their cholesterol level.

Clinical evidence states that there is insufficient evidence to identify which individuals benefit from taking aspirin for primary prevention.[4] Some people will suffer the adverse effect of bleeding while taking aspirin or be unable to tolerate it.

Control of hypertension is likely to reduce the risk of cardiovascular events with minimal adverse effects.[4]

Secondary prevention

Secondary prevention is the long-term management of people with a prior acute myocardial infarction or stroke or people at risk of ischaemic events. The lifestyle interventions useful in primary prevention will be helpful in secondary prevention too.

RAPID REFERRAL

You should be able to refer patients you suspect of having angina to a rapid access chest pain clinic so that a specialist can assess them within two weeks.

CARDIAC REHABILITATION

Cardiac rehabilitation can reduce the risk of death and further myocardial infarction. The programme provides advice and help on exercise, diet, stress and other aspects of getting back into full health following a heart attack. Patients can mix with others who are going through the same experience.[4,6]

MEDICATION

Patients are likely to be discharged from hospital on a cocktail of drugs. So review them and check that all are necessary and comply with local or national guidelines.

Antiplatelet medication such as low-dose aspirin (75 mg/day) reduces the risk of another episode of myocardial infarction, stroke or other vascular thrombosis. Benefits outweigh the risk of both cerebral and gastrointestinal haemorrhage. Other antiplatelet drugs, e.g. clopidogrel, are much more expensive and are usually only used if aspirin is contraindicated. Indigestion is the commonest side effect (and can somtimes be reduced by using enteric coated aspirin) and, in patients at high risk of bleeding, aspirin can be combined with a proton pump inhibitor.

Treatment with beta-blocking drugs reduces total mortality, sudden death and the risk of another myocardial infarction. No one type of beta-blocker is any better than another, so look for one with the lowest price that suits that patient. Remember that asthma is a contraindication to taking beta-blockers and about a quarter of people started on them suffer ill effects.[4]

Statins are the single most effective type of lipid lowering drugs for treatment to reduce cholesterol levels and reduce cardiovascular risk. Immediately after a myocardial infarction, a temporary reduction in cholesterol levels occurs, so measurement about 6 to 12 weeks after the event gives a better guide. Contraindications include liver disease and porphyria, so liver function should be checked before, within one to three months of starting treatment and then 6- to 12-monthly. Statins interact with other drugs broken down in the liver, macrolide antibiotics such as erythromycin and with grapefruit juice. The rare side-effect of myopathy should prompt discontinuation.

Angiotensin converting enzyme (ACE) inhibitors improve left ventricular function in patients who have had a myocardial infarction. Even without evidence of left ventricular dysfunction, outcomes in terms of fewer deaths, strokes and myocardial infarctions occur in patients given ACE inhibitors.[4] The once daily dose of the newer ACE inhibitors aids compliance.

In selected high-risk patients, anticoagulant therapy rather than aspirin may prevent further thrombotic episodes but are associated with a significant risk of haemorrhage.[4] Amiodarone may be required for control of tachyarrhythmias and reduces the risk of sudden death in this high-risk group of patients.[4]

Angina

People with stable angina should have appropriate investigations and treatment. Patients with angina will need nitrates. Glyceryl trinitrate tablets (that need renewing every eight weeks once opened) or a spray are most convenient for occasional use. Warn patients about potential side-effects, flushing, headache, etc. Consider longer acting preparations such as isosorbide mononitrate for more regular prophylaxis.

Patients with increasing frequency or severity of attacks should be referred urgently or as an emergency for consideration of revascularisation.[7]

Heart failure

There are specific standards for heart failure that include procedures for accurate diagnosis in suspected heart failure such as echocardiography. Identification of the cause, treatment of underlying conditions and treatment of heart failure should be offered. This domain is labelled as left ventricular dysfunction (LVD) in the quality and outcomes framework. Patients with suspected LVD should be treated with ACE inhibitors or angiotensin 2 receptor antagonists unless contraindications exist. These should be recorded.

What are the outcomes?

The overall aim is to reduce the incidence of coronary heart disease/coronary events (fatal and non-fatal), including myocardial infarction that comprise Standards 1 and 2 of the Coronary Heart Disease *NSF*.[5,6] Other standards in the *NSF* are recognised by points in the quality and outcomes framework.

Quality indicators in coronary heart disease

The quality points available are achievable on a sliding scale. Some of the quality indicators in coronary heart disease overlap with those for hypertension (*see* Table 10.2 overleaf).

Exception reporting is the same as for the quality targets for hypertension. That is, the patients do not wish to participate, have contraindications or unacceptable side-effects on medication, or have conditions making treatment inappropriate.

What are the challenges?

- Establishing an accurate and up-to-date register of all patients at risk is difficult. Practices that have only recently computerised or whose staff (clerical or health professionals) lack the skills to code the problems accurately and consistently have training needs that are difficult to meet in a busy general practice.
- It is often difficult to identify smokers and offer them advice about stopping, when they attend with their own set of problems that need to be met. The small numbers of people who succeed in stopping smoking (while worthwhile) can be discouraging.

Table 10.2:   Quality and outcomes measures for coronary heart disease

Criteria	Maximum thresholds (minimum 25%) (%)	Points
A register of patients with coronary heart disease	Practice prevalence in line with national/local prevalence figures	6
Patients with new onset angina referred for exercise testing or specialist assessment	90	7
Patients have their smoking status recorded in the last 15 months	90	7
Patients who smoke have been offered smoking cessation advice in the last 15 months	70	4
Patients have a blood pressure recorded in the last 15 months	90	7
Patients have a blood pressure on treatment of less than that recommended by the British Hypertension Society Guidelines (BP150/90) in the last 15 months	70	19
Patients have their cholesterol level recorded in the last 15 months	90	7
Patients have a cholesterol level on treatment of 5 mmol/l or less in the last 15 months	60	16
Patients are on antithrombotic therapy in the last 15 months	90	7
Patients are currently on a beta-blocker	50	7
Patients who have had a myocardial infarction are currently on an angiotensin converting enzyme inhibitor	70	7
Patients have received the influenza immunisation in the previous September to March	85	7
Subset for left ventricular dysfunction (LVD)		
The practice can produce a register of patients with CHD and LVD	As expected prevalence	4
The percentage of patients with a diagnosis of CHD and LVD (diagnosed after 1 April 2003) which has been confirmed by an echocardiogram	90	6
The percentage of patients with a diagnosis of CHD and LVD who are currently treated with ACE inhibitors (or A2 antagonists)	70	10

- Other lifestyle changes are also difficult to promote and sustain. The low level of success from weight reduction, dietary modification and increased physical activity is demotivating for health professionals inexperienced in health promotion activities.
- Delays in secondary care investigations and treatment prevent the best care from being offered. The delays prolong the inactivity and delay the return of patients to a productive and fully functional life. This increases the burden on staff working in primary care services who need to monitor and support patients more frequently and for longer periods.

What can you do to make it more likely that you will succeed?

- Identify what training needs practice teams have for accurate data entry and maintenance of disease registers. Lists of Read codes should be widely circulated in forms that are easily retrievable at the time of entry – either when a patient is consulting or when documents such as discharge letters are received.
- Practice teams need help to identify their patients accurately, capture those patients not currently on their systems and to ensure that those entered have correct diagnoses. This involves doing data searches for patients currently being prescribed commonly given cardiovascular medication such as nitrates and statins, as well as searching for diagnosis entries. Suitably trained clerical staff can do most of this work but confirmation of a patient's diagnosis, if not already recorded, requires medical input.
- Identifying key people who have responsibility for entering data received from other sources such as hospital letters, improves consistent and accurate data entry.
- Practice nurses trained in preventive interventions are more likely to ask and advise about lifestyle changes such as smoking, diet and exercise. Clerical staff can keep information up to date by entering information from forms completed by patients.
- Set up regular clinical audit to identify patients who have not been reviewed in the last 12 months. These patients can be invited, perhaps around their birthday to spread the workload, to a review appointment by one of the nurses. The use of a disease template, either on computer, or for later entry to computer, helps to ensure that all the relevant checks are made such as blood pressure, smoking history and advice or medication review. Ask the patients to have the relevant blood tests prior to the appointment, so that results are available at the time to aid decision making.
- Make sure that systems for referring to rapid access clinics are known and used. In one area, email referral to obtain an appointment within two weeks at the time of request was poorly used because of lack of understanding of how it might be operated by the referring GPs and clinicians' anxiety about using email.
- Feedback problems about investigation and treatment delays to the PCO for action.

Further reading

Chambers R, Wakley G and Iqbal Z (2001) *Cardiovascular Disease Matters in Primary Care.* Radcliffe Medical Press, Oxford.

Munafo M, Drury M, Wakley G *et al.* (2003) *Smoking Cessation Matters in Primary Care.* Radcliffe Medical Press, Oxford.

Wakley G, Chambers R and Ellis S (2004) *Demonstrating Your Competence 3: cardiovascular and neurological conditions.* Radcliffe Publishing, Oxford.

References

1 Third Joint Task Force of European and other Societies on Cardiovascular Disease Prevention in Clinical Practice (2003) European Guidelines on cardiovascular disease prevention in clinical practice. *European Journal of Cardiovascular Prevention and Rehabilitation.* **10(Suppl)**: S1–S78. www.escardio.org/NR/rdonlyres/A0EF5CA5-421B-45EF-A65C-19B9EC411261/0/CVD_Prevention_03_full.pdf

2 Joint Formulary Committee (2004) *British National Formulary.* British Medical Association and Royal Pharmaceutical Society, London. www.bnf.org

3 Foord-Kelcey (ed.) (2004) *Guidelines Vol. 23.* Medendium Group Publishing Ltd, Berkhampsted. www.eguidelines.co.uk

4 Godlee F (ed.) (2004) *Clinical Evidence.* BMJ Publishing Group, London. www.clinicalevidence.com

5 Department of Health (2000) *National Service Framework for Coronary Heart Disease.* Department of Health, London.

6 Chambers R, Wakley G and Iqbal Z (2001) *Cardiovascular Matters in Primary Care.* Radcliffe Medical Press, Oxford.

7 Department of Health (2003) *Delivering Better Heart Services: progress report.* Department of Health, London. www.dh.gov.uk/assetRoot/04/07/52/80/04075280.pdf

11

Stroke and transient ischaemic attack (TIA)

To explore how your primary care team might work together to improve the management of patients with stroke or TIA you can review a case (or cases) with which your team has been involved. You may prefer to use the two example cases at the start of this chapter. Read through them quickly before working on the problem case exercise (*see* page 157), or just photocopy Table 1.1 on page 7 to develop your own problem case. Include in your team people who will join in the problem-based learning discussion and be part of the solutions.

If you feel that you have insufficient knowledge to guide you in completing the problem-based learning, use the summary about stroke and TIA in the second part of this chapter and follow up the references if you need to learn more.

Example problem case 1

Problem Case:

A search set up for all patients with a diagnosis of stroke or TIA finds far more than would be expected from comparative data from the PCO's public health statistics. When separate searches are done on strokes, then on TIAs, the stroke numbers are below what would be expected and the number described as having had a TIA very much higher.

Who do you need in your team?

You might want a team that includes:

Patients and carers
Practice nurses
District nurses
Reception staff and secretaries
Practice manager
GPs
Nursing home staff.

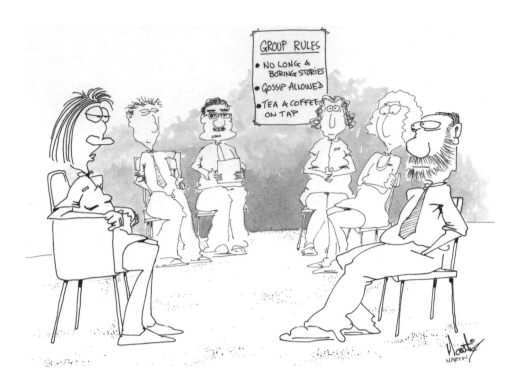

Where you are now

In the past many elderly patients with dizzy turns, unexplained falls or episodes of confusion tended to be labelled as having had TIAs. All of these labels will need to be reconsidered and recoded if not confirmed.

The data on strokes suggest that some patients have not had a stroke diagnosis correctly coded in their medical record.

What you do next

This might include.

- Deciding what to do about the label 'TIA'. It will be a lot of work to trawl through all the previous records. Most are likely to have inadequate data for a firm diagnosis. At a practice meeting it is agreed to code patients as G65 only when a diagnosis of TIA has been confirmed prospectively or when a patient is encountered who has a confirmed diagnosis.
- Setting up a system for screening hospital letters to code the diagnoses:
  - haemorrhagic stroke (Read code G61)
  - non-haemorrhagic stroke (G64)
  - stroke not otherwise specified (NOS) (G66)
  - TIA (G65)
- A search for patients on repeat prescriptions for antiplatelet drugs or warfarin is agreed. The patients identified are likely to be added to the coronary heart disease

register or left ventricular disease registers even if they are not eligible for the stroke register.

- Opportunistic coding of patients encountered during surgery or home consultations is encouraged.
- Informing patients, carers, nursing homes and district nurses about the purpose of the disease registers and encouraging them to enquire if patients have been added to the register.
- Completing Table 11.1.

What extra resources might this require?

- Time is scheduled for a practice meeting to discuss the diagnostic criteria for stroke and TIA and decide when to code the diagnosis of TIA.
- Time and training for all those involved in coding the diagnoses of stroke and TIA. You may need extra computer stations or an up-graded computer system for the additional recording work that needs to be done. Extra staff time will be needed for work to be completed.
- Designated person to carry out a search for patients on repeat prescriptions for antiplatelet drugs or warfarin. Additional people may need training in setting up searches as the number and frequency are likely to increase. Trained staff need protected time to add any patients to the correct registers.
- Anyone who encounters patients with stroke or TIA requires training on the agreed codes and how they should be entered. Staff who do not usually enter data, such as district nurses or a non-computer-literate GP, may need training and access, if this is useful for them and the practice, or a designated person who can do this for them.
- Designated member of the team needs time to prepare information, posters and to train reception staff to answer queries from patients and carers about registers and confidentiality.

The outcomes

These might include.

- The stroke register becoming more complete and accurate.
- Everyone having the information to code diagnoses of stroke and TIA correctly for the future.
- Diagnosis on letters about patients seen in secondary care being coded correctly and recorded in the medical records.
- Patients being recalled for an annual review.
- Patients understanding the purpose of the register and that of the annual review.

How would you demonstrate that you have achieved your outcomes?

A comparison between the proportion of patients on the register with a diagnosis of stroke or TIA is roughly similar to that expected by the public health data supplied by the PCO.

Table 11.1:   Role and responsibilities checklist – *for each task tick the box for each team member who has a role or responsibility – then note your role and responsibilities for the task*

Completed by: _____

Task	Primary care team member							What are your roles and your responsibilities?
	Doctor	*Practice nurse*	*District nurse*	*Reception team*	*Practice manager*	*Nursing home staff*	*Other*	
Identifying patients who should be included on the register	✔	✔	✔	✔	✔	✔	✔	*e.g. Making sure that people suspected but not confirmed, of having the condition are **not** included on the register*
Task 2								
Task 3								
Task 4								
Task 5								

Example problem case 2

Problem Case:

A computer template for the annual review of patients who have had a stroke or TIA is completed by the practice nurse carrying out the review. However, when patients are reviewed by GPs or district nurses, the template is not completed and data is often missing.

Who do you need in your team?

You might want a team that includes:

Patients and carers
Practice nurses
District nurses
GPs
Computer-trained staff
Healthcare assistants
Phlebotomists
Practice manager.

Where you are now

The practice nurses do most of the annual checks together with data collection by the healthcare assistants. The healthcare assistants ask about smoking and aspirin use, and record blood pressures. The practice nurses take blood for fasting cholesterol level and any other blood tests such as liver function, electrolytes and urea. They give smoking cessation advice and review the patient's daily living function and capabilities. Practice nurses often find that patients combine the review with a visit for an influenza immunisation or turn up at the 'flu clinic with their friends. The district nurses are willing to do annual checks on patients they visit at home, but have no access to the computer terminals in the practice. The GPs carry out reviews on those patients who have raised blood pressure or cholesterol readings, or additional medical conditions.

What you do next

The practice manager arranges a practice meeting with lunch provided and a short interactive presentation from an occupational therapist about what help she can offer to patients who have had a stroke. This is followed by a (non-accusatory) discussion about the lack of data being recorded by the GPs and district nurses when reviews are carried out.

You decide that all patients will have a designated date for review between April and September, i.e. not when 'flu immunisations are being done. They will be called according to the letter of alphabet of their surname, e.g. A–D in April, E–H in May, etc. At this review date the healthcare assistant will collect all the data and the phlebotomist will collect the blood samples. The data on patients who are house-bound will be entered on to a paper form by the phlebotomist who does home blood tests and given to the healthcare assistant for entering on to the electronic medical record. Patients are supplied with information about smoking cessation services where appropriate and this is recorded. A template on daily living activities is completed. If any unmet needs are identified, the healthcare assistant refers to the practice nurse or GP.

Maximal efforts to review and record data will be made for the group of patients who are also on other registers such as diabetes, coronary heart disease or hypertension.

Clinical activities will be recorded separately, informed by the data already collected.

What extra resources might this require?

- Extra training for the healthcare assistants.
- An additional healthcare assistant is recruited and trained.
- The phlebotomist has an extra session a week.
- A practice nurse is identified as supervisor for the activities of the healthcare assistants.
- As more needs are identified, additional services from occupational therapists, speech therapists and physiotherapists are likely to be required.
- Influenza sessions are designated as immunisation sessions only.

The outcomes

These might include.

- Consistent review of medical and social needs.
- Consistent and reliable capture of data.
- Patients having a 'one-stop review' unless complex needs are identified that require further input or assessment.
- Influenza sessions are not disrupted by requests for routine blood pressure recording or other data collection.

How would you demonstrate that you have achieved your outcomes?

Searches for data recording demonstrate improved and consistent data collection.

Problem case exercise

Problem Case:

A practice protocol includes rapid referral to a TIA clinic for patients suffering minor strokes or suspected TIAs who do not require hospital admission. However, the waiting list for this clinic is now several weeks. The delay for computerised tomography (CT) or magnetic resonance imaging (MRI) scan for people with a diagnosis of minor stroke is several months.

Who do you need in your team?

Where you are now

What you do next

Continued

What extra resources might this require?

The outcomes

How would you demonstrate that you have achieved your outcomes?

Why stroke and transient ischaemic attack (TIA) are important

Stroke is the third most common cause of death in most developed countries. Strokes can occur at any age but half of all strokes happen in people over the age of 70 years. About a third of people with acute ischaemic attacks (a 'brain attack') die within a month. Of those who survive, about half still have some level of disability after six months.[1] The risk of further attacks or a stroke is very high (10 to 20% in the next six months).[2]

What are strokes and TIAs?

A stroke has rapidly developing clinical symptoms and signs of focal or global loss of cerebral function lasting more than 24 hours, if death does not occur. No other cause apart from vascular insufficiency is involved. About 80% of all acute strokes are ischaemic, usually as the result of a clot or an embolus blocking a blood vessel. Subarachnoid or an intracerebral bleed cause the remainder. A TIA lasts less than 24 hours with complete or almost complete recovery.

Atherosclerosis is the common underlying condition associated with stroke in older people. Risk factors include hypertension, diabetes, smoking, high levels of low-density lipoprotein, cholesterol, obesity and inactivity. Other conditions that increase the risk of stroke include those where thrombosis, embolus or vasculitis is more likely.

What should you do, when and how?

Primary prevention

Primary prevention of strokes and TIAs targets underlying conditions. Prevention of cardiovascular disease will also help to prevent cerebrovascular disease.

The *National Service Framework for Older People*[3] for England states that by April 2004 primary care trusts will ensure that:

*   all practices use protocols agreed with local experts to treat and identify patients at risk of stroke
*   all GP practices have an agreed protocol for rapid referral for TIA
*   all GP practices can identify patients who have had a stroke and are caring for them according to agreed protocols
*   every general practice has established clinical audit systems for stroke.

It also requires that all hospitals looking after patients with a stroke will have a specialised service as described in the stroke service model.

Regard the development of symptoms and signs of a stroke as an emergency, similar to that of a heart attack. Calling strokes 'brain attacks' as the Stroke Association suggests might help to focus everyone's attention on the need for urgent action.[4] Refer to hospital with the expectation that a patient with persisting symptoms is admitted to the nearest stroke unit. Brain imaging should be carried out as soon as possible, at least within 24 hours and more urgently if there is any suspicion of a bleed or an alternative diagnosis.

Patients with symptoms of a TIA with a good immediate recovery should be referred urgently and you should expect them to be seen within seven days (the new recommendations).[2] While waiting for assessment, give 300 mg aspirin immediately (or alternative antiplatelet medication if aspirin is contraindicated) unless there is any suspicion of a bleed, and treat any hypertension.

Specialist stroke services can be provided in the community as effectively as in hospital, once the patient has been stabilised and has recovered sufficiently to be able to transfer from bed to a chair. Good information for patients and carers is essential and the Royal College of Physicians has updated the patient and carers' information booklet in line with their latest guidelines.[5] You should expect specialist stroke services to:

*   screen for depression and anxiety within a month and keep the patient's mood under review

- screen for cognitive impairment
- arrange an assessment for intensive speech and language therapy if aphasia is present
- have a physiotherapist who has expertise in neuro-disability to provide co-ordinated therapy for physical disability
- arrange assessment by an occupational therapist with specialist knowledge in neurological rehabilitation if the patient has difficulties in daily living activities
- assess the need for equipment or adaptations to increase independence
- assess whether pain is a significant problem and refer to a specialised service if necessary.

Secondary prevention

Secondary prevention aims to reduce the risk of further strokes. The stroke team should draw up and implement an individual plan within seven days of the onset of the attack. Give all patients advice on lifestyle modification as for primary prevention of cardiovascular disease.[1] Hypertension persisting after two weeks should be treated according to British Hypertension Society standards.[6] If patients are not on anti-coagulants, give aspirin or other antiplatelet agents and a statin if the total choles-terol is above 3.5 mmol/l, unless there are contraindications to therapy. Patients who have a stroke in the carotid artery territory should be considered for carotid endarterectomy as soon as they are fit for surgery, preferably within two weeks of a TIA. Symptoms and signs in the carotid artery territory might include any of the following.

- Hemiparesis (confined to one side of the body).
- Hemisensory syndrome (face, arm and leg on one side of the body).
- Dysphasia (affecting language, not articulation).
- Visuospatial neglect (no knowledge of one side of the visual field and appearing to ignore visual and spatial cues coming from that direction).
- Visual loss confined to one eye.

Ischaemia in the posterior circulation is suggested by:

- diplopia (seeing two images)
- vertigo (rotatory or tilting dizziness)
- nausea
- complete loss of vision or homonimous hemianopia (loss of corresponding halves of the one side of the field of vision in both eyes)
- crossed motor or crossed sensory syndrome (involving the face on one side and the leg and/or arm on the other side).

The longer term management of patients should include a plan involving patients and carers so that all necessary equipment and support services are in place before discharge from hospital. Continuing treatment should start without any delay after discharge and patients and carers should have information about local services. Independence is encouraged but arrangements for review of the patient's needs and further access to rehabilitation should be available.

What are the outcomes?

The key issues are survival and the ability to perform daily activities and to fulfil social roles. Options for measuring longer term outcomes include measures of quality of life (for example, in the form of multi-dimensional health profiles such as the SF–36, the Nottingham Health Profile or the EuroQol) and global handicap (for example, using the modified Rankin Scale, the Functional Autonomy Measurement Scale, the Edinburgh Rehabilitation Scale, and the London Handicap Scale).[6] Alternatively, individual components of handicap can be measured. These include long-term disability, mental health and functioning, economic self-sufficiency and social integration. At a minimum, measurement should occur at six months and subsequently every year.[6]

Quality indicators for the care of stroke and TIA

The quality points available under the GMS contract are achievable on a sliding scale and this domain overlaps with CHD, diabetes, asthma and chronic obstructive pulmonary disease (COPD) – *see* Table 11.2.

Exception reporting will be the same as for coronary heart disease, so make sure that you record your discussions with patients.

What are the challenges?

- Lack of recognition of the urgency of the condition both by the public and to a lesser degree by health professionals.
- Lack of resources and shortage of people to put into action the guidelines for care.

What can you do to make it more likely that you will succeed?

- Invest in research and take steps to put existing findings into practice. This will benefit all those affected by stroke.
- Introduce stroke prevention programmes. This will substantially reduce needless death and disability each year due to stroke.
- A lead primary care stroke clinician at a local level would be able to shape services around the needs of the patient and bring about improvements to community health care.
- End the postcode lottery of care for stroke patients – everybody who has a stroke should receive assessment and care in a stroke unit.

Table 11.2:   Quality and outcomes measures for stroke and TIA

Criteria	Maximum thresholds (minimum 25%) (%)	Points
The practice can produce a register of patients with stroke or TIA	Compatible with expected prevalence	4
Percentage of new patients with a presumptive diagnosis of stroke after 1 April 2003 who have been referred for confirmation of diagnosis by CT or MRI scan	80	2
All patients on the stroke and TIA register have a record of their smoking status recorded in the last 15 months	90	3
Patients on the stroke and TIA register who smoke have a record that smoking cessation advice has been offered in the last 15 months	70	2
Patients on the stroke and TIA register have a record of their blood pressure in the last 15 months	90	2
Patients on the stroke and TIA register have a record of their total cholesterol in the last 15 months	90	2
Treatment with aspirin/other platelet or an anticoagulant is recorded for patients who have a confirmed non-haemorrhagic stroke or TIA	90	4
Patients on the stroke and TIA register have a record of having had influenza immunisation in the preceding September to March	85	2
Patients on the stroke and TIA register have a record of their blood pressure at 150/90 or below in the last 15 months	70	5
Patients on the stroke and TIA register have a record of their total cholesterol at 5 mmol/l or less in the last 15 months	60	5

Further reading

Wakley G, Chambers R and Ellis S (2004) *Demonstrating Your Competence 3: cardiovascular and neurological conditions.* Radcliffe Publishing, Oxford.

References

1　Godlee F (ed.) (2004) *Clinical Evidence Concise. Issue 11.* BMJ Publishing Group, London and www.clinicalevidence.com

2　www.rcplondon.ac.uk/pubs/books/stroke/stroke_conciseguide_2ed.pdf

3　Philp I and Platt D (co-chairmen External Reference Group) (2001) *National Service Framework for Older People.* Department of Health, London.

4　www.stroke.org.uk Tel: 0845 30 33 100 for details of local contacts.

5　Intercollegiate Stroke Working Party (2004) *National Clinical Guidelines for Stroke.* Royal College of Physicians, London. www.rcplondon.ac.uk/pubs/books/stroke/stroke_patientcarer_2ed.pdf

6　www.leeds.ac.uk/nuffield/infoservices/UKCH/stroke.html

12

Medicines management

Medicines management is 'the systematic provision of medicines therapy, through a partnership of effort between patients and professionals, to deliver best patient outcomes at minimised cost'.[1] This definition implies new relationships of partnership between the pharmacist, the patient and the primary care team.

Medicines management can bring teamwork to primary care like no other concept. There are roles for staff of all skill backgrounds. The key to success is realising the potential of medicines management and implementing best practice together as a team. The advent of nurse specialists, GPs with special interests, and highly skilled pharmacists looks set to reorient the management of people with chronic disease, increasing the capacity of primary care and raising the threshold for hospital referral. Good skill mix allows highly skilled clinicians to devote their time to more complex clinical tasks, while other team members progress their competencies and capabilities in new roles. Patients benefit through a reduced chance of errors, medication regimes optimised to their clinical needs and increased convenience.

To explore how your primary care team might work together to improve medicines management you can review a case (or cases) with which your team has been involved. You may prefer to use the two example cases at the start of this chapter. Read through them quickly before working on the problem case exercise (*see* page 170), or just photocopy Table 1.1 on page 7 to develop your own problem case. Include in your team people who will join in the problem-based learning discussion and be part of the solutions.

If you feel that you have insufficient knowledge to guide you in completing the problem-based learning, use the summary about medicines management in the second part of this chapter and follow up the references if you need to learn more.

Example problem case 1

Problem Case:

A baseline audit of the practice computer system at Pointless Surgery shows that achievement against the quality and outcomes target of 'medication review for all those on four or more medicines' has not been met. The target is for 80% of patients to have a medication review recorded in the last 15 months.

Who do you need in your team?

You might want a team that includes:

Reception staff – producing and distributing repeat prescriptions
Nurses and doctors – whenever they spot patients on four or more medicines
Practice or community pharmacist input – identifying patients for review. Perhaps conducting reviews within a defined structure
Practice manager – assessing audit results, identifying patients for review.

Where you are now

Analysis of the patients without Read codes for medication review shows a pattern. Patients over 75 years, people with diabetes and those with asthma seem to have missed out on medication reviews, according to the Read coding. You realise that the absence of patients over 75 years is due to Dr S, who reviews those on four or more medicines every six months, in line with the NSF for the elderly. Sister N, the practice nurse specialist, runs regular diabetes and asthma clinics when patients are coded after their appointment. This suggests that Dr S does not use Read codes (or uses unrecognised codes) when consulting. Patients being reviewed by Sister N for diabetes or asthma are not being recorded as having had a medication review, although she is coding other information.

What you do next

This might include.

- Convening a practice meeting to discuss who records medication reviews, how and where.
- Looking at the literature encompassing medication review strategies.
- Assessing how you conduct medication reviews as a team. Could this be made more efficient?
- Contacting your PCO's prescribing adviser to ask them which Read codes will be accepted for GP contract purposes. Could they provide extra pharmacist/nurse support to conduct reviews?
- Asking community pharmacists to refer those perceived to be in need of review to one of the GPs in the practice.
- Asking reception staff to bring to patients' attention that they need a review.
- Asking patients themselves to book themselves in for a medication review, via a message on their repeat medication counterfoil.
- Looking at the repeat medication controls on the prescribing system. Does it flag up those requiring review? Can it be overridden, and if so, how many times and by whom?
- Putting in place a regular audit to pick up people on a disease register who have not been reviewed and inviting them in.
- Completing Table 12.1.

What extra resources might this require?

- Time and resources for a staff meeting.
- Time to look at and evaluate the literature.

- Time and skills to develop a review framework, for example, is it just a blood pressure check they need?
- Time to conduct the extra reviews.
- Time and skills to train appropriate staff in the area of medication review.
- Extra practice pharmacist or specialist nurse input, perhaps sourced by the PCO.
- Time for collaboration with local community pharmacists.
- Time to contact your IT supplier regarding system controls for your practice computer.
- Clerical time for audit.

The outcomes

These might include.

- Achievement of the quality and outcomes target
- Increased patient safety
- Increased cost-effectiveness
- Increased process efficiency
- Increased patient satisfaction
- Increased staff satisfaction.

How would you demonstrate that you have achieved your outcomes?

- Repeat audit at intervals to measure your progress towards the targets.
- Audit the occurrence of any critical events.
- Assess patient satisfaction – via a practice questionnaire.
- Get feedback from staff at subsequent practice meetings.

Example problem case 2

> **Problem Case:**
>
> The PCO prescribing incentive scheme has just landed on your desk. This year's scheme is 'designed to supplement the new contract and tackle local prescribing issues'. As a practice, you choose reduction of antibiotic prescribing as your key target.

Who do you need in your team?

You might want a team that includes:

Reception staff – strategy awareness
Practice nurses – particularly if involved in triage
Health visitors, midwives and district nurses
Community pharmacists, to ensure they advise patients about antibiotics appropriately

Table 12.1:   Role and responsibilities checklist – *for each task tick the box for each team member who has a role or responsibility – then note your role and responsibilities for the task*

Completed by: _____

| Task | Primary care team member | | | | | | | What are your roles and your responsibilities? |
	Doctor	Practice nurse	Local pharmacist	Reception team	Practice manager	Other	Other	
Agree how medication reviews are conducted (who, codes, etc.)	✔	✔	✔	✔	✔	✔	✔	*e.g. Making sure that I use correct Read code for medication review*
Task 2								
Task 3								
Task 4								
Task 5								

GPs – deciding the clinical merits of antibiotics
Practice manager, when dealing with complaints!

Where you are now

Looking at your prescribing data with the prescribing adviser at your annual meeting, you concede that improvements could be made to antibiotic prescribing. You acknowledge that there are both patient and clinical education issues.

What you do next

This might include.

- Looking at the literature regarding appropriate antibiotic prescribing.
- Evaluating which strategies other practices/PCOs have used to educate patients about antibiotics.
- Arranging a practice meeting, trying to involve the wider healthcare team – community pharmacists, district nurses, health visitors and midwives if possible. Consider inviting patients along too to gauge their opinions. Draft and agree a practice formulary so that all GPs offer the same advice and take the same approach to prescribing.
- Asking the prescribing adviser/practice pharmacist to contribute to, or peer review the draft practice formulary; assess the types of antibiotic used in your practice and how these compare to local and national standards.
- Finalising practice formulary and sharing with the practice team and local pharmacists.
- Setting an audit date to check progress.

What extra resources might this require?

- Time to look at and evaluate the literature.
- Time to communicate with other organisations who have tried similar strategies.
- Clerical time to arrange a mutually convenient meeting to try to ensure the widest participation.
- Time to discuss prescribing data with prescribing adviser or practice pharmacist.
- Time for collaboration with local community pharmacists.
- Clinical time to assess the applicability of any formulary available.
- Clerical time for audit.

The outcomes

These might include.

- Less doctor dependence for minor ailments with pharmacists more involved in advising and treating minor ailments.
- Improved patient safety and concordance or compliance.
- Cost-effective, evidence-based use of antibiotics.
- Rewards via the prescribing incentive scheme.

How would you demonstrate that you have achieved your outcomes?

• Audit re-attendance of patients for antibiotics.
• Comparison of prescribing data before and after implementation of your action plan.

Problem case exercise

Problem Case:

Last month, you adopted the 'advanced access' appointments system. Bookings are made on the day of the necessary appointment. You also take repeat prescription orders over the phone. You reinstated this telephone service recently in response to your practice patients' suggestions. The receptionist taking the call checks the computer records at the same time to minimise the possibility of errors being made by verbal requests for prescriptions. Patients are starting to grumble that they cannot get through on the telephone to either book an appointment or request a prescription. You add the issue about telephone access to the agenda of the next practice meeting.

Who do you need in your team?

Where you are now

What you do next

Continued

What extra resources might this require?

The outcomes

How would you demonstrate that you have achieved your outcomes?

Why medicines management is important

Around 20% of PCO funds are spent on medicines and medicines services.[2] Up to 50% of people cannot, or do not, take their medicines as prescribed.[3] In the period 1997 to 2002 costs of prescribing increased by 57% (*see* Figure 12.1).[4] These costs are likely to continue to increase as chronic disease management is improved and patients live longer. *Help the Aged* estimates that by 2025, a quarter of Britons will be over 60 years and half of those will be over 75 years old. Most people over 75 years take one or more regular medications, and almost 40% take four or more.[3]

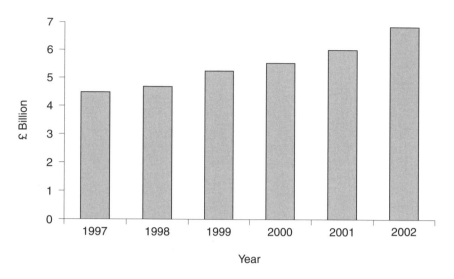

Figure 12.1: Annual cost of prescriptions, England 1997 to 2002. (Data from *Health and Personal Social Services Statistics*, Department of Health.[4])

Increasing polypharmacy creates risks: the majority of patients benefit from their medicines, but some do not. More than £100m of medicines are returned to pharmacies each year and it is likely that this figure is only the tip of the iceberg of drugs not ingested.[5] Medication is implicated in between 5 and 17% of hospital admissions.[3] A study of repeat prescribing across 50 practices in Leeds found that 72% of repeat prescriptions had not been reviewed in the previous 15 months.[6]

Pharmacy in the Future set a target for all primary care teams to have medicines management services in place by April 2004.[5] A survey in June 2004 showed that progress had been made as pockets of good practice, but not as a uniform improvement.[7]

Concordance and patient empowerment in medicines management

Concordance and patient empowerment are key ideals in clinical practice and they punctuate guidelines promoting good chronic disease management. Most patients have the capacity to contribute to decisions regarding their care. Unnecessary ill health and waste of resources stem from patients who are not involved and do not understand their treatment. This is particularly important now that many patients live with medical conditions for a large proportion of their lives. Patients who understand their medicines can self-manage many aspects of their treatment and help themselves.

The Expert Patient Programme teaches patients to manage their own long-term conditions and is a good example of the on-going shift in the doctor–patient (or nurse–patient) relationship.[8] Concerned with the wider issues surrounding concordance, the Medicines Partnership promotes patient involvement and provides learning resources for clinicians.[9] There is ever increasing access to information, and signposting patients to simple and reliable sources can allow them to answer a lot of their own questions, at their own convenience. By encouraging patients to monitor their own progress and understand the consequences of their lifestyles, outcomes are improved and stresses on healthcare resources are decreased.

What is medicines management?

Medicines management can be defined as 'a system of processes and behaviours that determines how medicines are used by patients and the NHS'.[2] Broadly you can separate this into patient-centred clinical interventions, and system and process interventions.

Patient-centred interventions

Activities include:

* medication review clinics
* domiciliary medication reviews
* specialised disease management clinics.

System and process interventions

Activities include:

* repeat prescribing control
* management of communication at healthcare interfaces.

Who should do it, how do we do it, who should we target?

Skill mix and implementation

Every practice has a different mix of patient demographics and staff skills. The initial step to rationalising something you probably do already, is to take stock of who you have and what they can, and are willing to do. By ensuring correct use of skills throughout the practice, you can free up the time of key clinicians. Key to your success is implementing a range of measures that integrate with processes already in place. For example the practice with a nurse specialist may just need to ensure that they are Read coding medicines management interventions appropriately, for patients within their clinical specialty. In another practice, a specialist pharmacist may come in and review patients from selected groups, or review patients in their own homes. As a GP, you may allocate specific appointments for medication review. Everyone will benefit if your clerical and managerial staff can also be involved, for example, through improved monitoring of the repeat prescribing system.

The medication review 'clinic'

Medication review has been defined as 'a structured, critical examination of a patient's medicines with the objective of reaching an agreement with the patient about treatment, optimising the impact of medicines, minimising the number of medication-related problems and reducing waste'.[10]

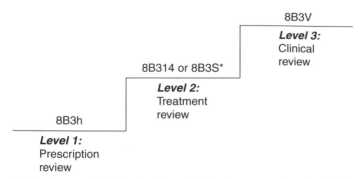

*Not all systems recognise Read codes with more than four characters; use the option of '8B3S'.

Figure 12.2: Structure for a medication review strategy. (Adapted from *Room for Review*.[10])

A good medication review strategy can prevent an important task becoming an unmanageable burden on clinical time. The right people should get the right type of review at the right time, from the right people. Figure 12.2 suggests a structure that could be implemented and Table 12.2 summarises possible details.

Structured reviews facilitate the attainment of many targets outside of the medicines management indicator, particularly within the clinical section of the quality and outcomes framework (*see* Tables 12.3 and 12.4).

Medication review can also be a good time for a general patient check, to update recorded data and achieve more quality points. Those invited in specifically may not be regular attendees and such information may help trigger further healthcare interventions. A 'health check' questionnaire could be handed to patients when booking in to be completed whilst waiting to be seen to obtain useful data such as smoking and influenza/pneumoccocal immunisation status or frequency/date of last seizure if the patient has epilepsy.

Table 12.2: Three levels for a medication review (adapted from *Room for Review*[10])

	Read code	Patient present	Basic outline	By whom?
Level 1	8B3h	No	Basic 'housekeeping' such as optimising doses, deleting old items, synchronising quantities	Clerical staff, including via a pharmacy intervention scheme
Level 2	8B314 or 8B3S*	No	Treatment review – a clinical and cost-effectiveness review with full access to patient records	Doctor, nurse, pharmacist
Level 3	8B3V	Yes	Clinical medication review – as above but with patient and any necessary laboratory results	Doctor, nurse, pharmacist

*Not all systems recognise Read codes with more than four characters; use the option of '8B3S'.

Table 12.3:   Quality and outcomes measures for medicines management

Criteria	Maximum thresholds (minimum 25%) (%)	Points
Medicines Management 5 A medication review is recorded in the notes in the preceding 15 months for all patients being prescribed four or more repeat medicines	80	7
Medicines Management 9 A medication review is recorded in the notes in the preceding 15 months for all patients being prescribed repeat medicines	80	8
Records 9 For repeat medicines, an indication for the drug can be identified in the records for drugs added to repeat prescription (with effect from 1 April 2004)	80	4
Records 7 The medicines that a patient is receiving are clearly listed in his or her record	No threshold	1

Table 12.4:   Quality and outcomes measures for medication review within clinical indicators

Criteria	Maximum thresholds (minimum 25%) (%)	Points
COPD 7 The percentage of patients with COPD receiving inhaled treatment in whom there is a record that inhaler technique has been checked in the preceding two years	90	6
Epilepsy 3 The percentage of patients age 16 years and over on drug treatment for epilepsy who have a record of medication review in the previous 15 months	90	4
Mental Health 2 The percentage of patients with severe long-term mental health problems with a review recorded in the preceding 15 months	90	23

Domiciliary medication review

Visiting patients at home, primarily the elderly/housebound can give valuable insights into how a patient's computer record, particularly their use of medicines, translates into 'real life'. To aid with these reviews, some areas have created domiciliary pharmacist visiting schemes, though evidence has shown that many have demised through lack of referrals. Only 17% of PCOs had such schemes in place in one report.[11]

Strategies such as the Single Assessment Process are likely to trigger requests for medication reviews more often, particularly in the domiciliary setting. It is likely that PCOs will support existing domiciliary visiting schemes (whoever is the provider) and perhaps commission new ones as the demand for this type of service increases.

Specialised disease management clinics

These clinics are now being routinely provided by general practitioners with special interests, nurse specialists and in some areas, by practice pharmacists. A problem presented by the GMS contract has been the definition of a medication review. For example, will patients attending for a review of their asthma with the practice nurse, where review of their treatment is a part, be considered as having been reviewed from the perspective of medicines management targets? This is particularly complicated if there are co-existing conditions that the specialist cannot, or does not review at the same time.

Repeat prescribing control

A robust repeat prescribing system is crucial to good medicines management. It should result in:

- identification of patients requiring clinical review
- increased patient satisfaction
- minimisation of mis-direction/abuse of prescription medicines
- improved patient safety
- reduced waste
- decreased GP workload.

There are specific targets in relation to repeat prescribing in the medicines management indicator of the GMS contract as Table 12.5 describes. The National Prescribing Centre has produced a comprehensive resource detailing good practice in repeat prescribing.[12]

Management of communication at healthcare interfaces

Threats to continuity of patient care at healthcare interfaces is all too common a problem and is often complicated by medication. Strategies implemented by hospitals such as use of patients' own drugs and 28-day prescribing on discharge are examples of good medicines management in secondary care. Their implementation has meant that waste is reduced on admission and convenience for both GP and patient is increased on discharge. Problems with illegible or non-existent discharge letters are still encountered in primary care but can be reduced by good communication and in the future, by electronic patient records.

Table 12.5:   Quality and outcomes measures in relation to repeat prescribing

Criteria	Points
Medicines Management 4	3
The number of hours from requesting a prescription to availability for collection by the patient is 72 hours or less (excluding weekends and bank/local holidays)	
Medicines Management 8	6
The number of hours from requesting a prescription to availability for collection by the patient is 48 hours or less (excluding weekends and bank/local holidays)	
Education 4	3
All new staff receive induction training	

Who to target

Medicines management is multi-faceted and needs to be tackled on two levels – that of the patient and that of the process. From the perspective of the patient, ideally involve anyone having regular medication, though in your climate of priorities, you first need to look where most benefits will be achieved. Once you realise that the elderly and people with chronic diseases consume the most medication, it is rational to target elderly people with chronic conditions, managed by medication, amongst your patient population. With the quality and outcomes framework in mind, first work through patients within the clinical indicator groups, unless these are already provided for.

What are the outcomes?

You should aim to:

- increase the number of patients receiving medication reviews
- increase the 'level' of reviews used, ideally to level 3 annually
- ensure that Read codes and your medication review structure are in line with national or local guidance
- provide education to patients about their conditions or medication regimens, to aid their self-management
- improve the cost-effectiveness (not necessarily reduce the cost) of prescribing
- improve patient satisfaction, through increased efficiency and improved treatment.

What are the challenges?

- Structuring review and repeat prescribing processes and balancing skill mix to ensure enough capacity.
- Recalling patients who consider themselves well and without need for medical intervention. Remember to exception report those who consistently fail to attend for review when invited.
- Encouraging patients to learn about their conditions and medication and act accordingly.
- Overcoming resistance to change from staff who are happy in their present roles.

What can you do to make it more likely that you will succeed?

- Promote teamworking. Staff are more likely to expand their current roles. The practice is also more likely to attract highly skilled staff such as nurse specialists and GPs with special interests.
- Make the most of the skills you have in the practice currently and what can be 'commissioned' externally. The emergence of a new contract for pharmacy is likely to see expanded roles for more pharmacists, particularly in areas such as medication review.
- Implement a robust repeat prescribing policy, ensuring all staff are trained in their roles.
- Make sure that there is a regular audit cycle to monitor progress and provide motivation for staff.
- Give the practice questionnaire to patients to gain feedback on developments. Incorporate patient opinion into the way the practice runs.

Improving medicines management should be everyone's business.[13] Many patients receive less than optimal care if they find their medicines difficult to take or hard to remember or when they have complicated regimes involving several different drugs which are not reviewed often or well enough. Good medicines management is dependent upon teamwork and a holistic approach to care that engages with patients and carers as partners.

References

1   Tweedie A (2002) Medicines management and change management – the PSNC pilot trials. *Pharmaceutical Journal.* **268**: 146. www.pharmj.com/pdf/articles/pj_20020202_ psncpilot.pdf

2   National Prescribing Centre (2002) *Medicines management services – why are they important?* NPC, Liverpool. www.npc.co.uk/MeReC_Bulletins/2001Volumes/pdfs/vol12no6.pdf

3   Department of Health (2001) *Medicines and Older People: implementing medicines-related aspects of the NSF for older people.* Department of Health, London. www.dh.gov.uk

4   Department of Health (2004) *Health and Personal Social Services Statistics.* Department of Health, London. www.performance.doh.gov.uk/HPSSS/

5   Department of Health (2000) *Pharmacy in the future: implementing the NHS Plan.* Department of Health, London. www.dh.gov.uk/

6   Zermansky AG (1996) Who controls repeats? *British Journal of General Practice.* **46**: 643–7.

7   National Prescribing Centre (2004) *Survey of Medicines Management Activity in PCTs.* NPC, Liverpool. www.npc.co.uk/mms/Web_Dev/Extras/primary_care_survey_june_2004.pdf

8   Department of Health (2001) *The Expert Patient – a new approach to chronic disease management for the 21st century.* Department of Health, London. www.expertpatients.nhs.uk

9   The Medicines Partnership (2004). www.concordance.org/

10   The Medicines Partnership (2002) *Room for Review: a guide to medication review.* The Medicines Partnership, London. www.medicines-partnership.org/medication-review/ room-for-review

11   Bhattacharya D, Wright DJ and Purvis JR (2003) Pharmacist domiciliary visiting: review of English services. *International Journal of Pharmacy Practice.* **11**: 8. www.pharmj.com/ IJPP/bpc2003/ijpp_bpc2003_r08.pdf

12 National Prescribing Centre (2004) *Saving Time, Helping Patients: a good practice guide to quality repeat prescribing.* NPC, Liverpool. www.npc.co.uk/repeat_prescribing/pdf/repeat_ prescribing_document1.pdf

13 Department of Health (2004) *Management of Medicines.* Department of Health, London.

13

Chronic obstructive pulmonary disease (COPD)

To explore how your primary care team might work together to improve the management of patients with COPD you can review a case (or cases) with which your team has been involved. You may prefer to use the two example cases at the start of this chapter. Read through them quickly before working on the problem case exercise (*see* page 187), or just photocopy Table 1.1 on page 7 to develop your own problem case. Include in your team people who will join in the problem-based learning discussion and be part of the solutions.

If you feel that you have insufficient knowledge to guide you in completing the problem-based learning, use the summary about COPD in the second part of this chapter and follow up the references if you need to learn more.

Example problem case 1

Problem Case:

One of the receptionists has taken on the task of sending out invitations and recording the data for influenza immunisation.[1] She has recently done the European Computer Driving Licence qualification and is keen to use her skills. She and the practice manager have changed her job description and grading to recognise her new skills. She spends time reconciling all the people drawn from various categories – over 65 years, on the asthma, COPD, or CHD registers, etc., so that no one receives duplicate invitations. She records and excludes from invitation anyone with a recorded allergy or adverse reaction to influenza immunisation. She attends immunisation sessions with the practice nurse and records all the immunisations. She tells the practice manager that she has had several irate phone calls from patients who have been sent a second reminder invitation when they have already had the immunisation or do not want it. She is concerned that others in the team may be un-cooperative because they resent her new role.

Who do you need in your team?

You might want a team that includes:

Reception staff
Practice manager
Practice nurses
District nurses
GPs
Patients and carers
Pharmacists
Nursing home staff.

Where you are now

An investigation by the practice manager identifies several data collection problems.

- Some GPs have been giving the immunisation opportunistically to those who ask for it either when they attend surgery or on home visits.
- District nurses have been giving influenza immunisation to some of the patients that they visit as they did last year.
- A pharmacy on the edge of the practice area is offering influenza immunisation to anyone who wants it.
- One large nursing home, that has patients registered with several practices, has decided to immunise all staff and patients themselves after problems with co-ordination of immunisations in previous years.
- Messages from patients declining immunisation are not being recorded and passed on.

What you do next

This might include.

- A practice meeting to which the pharmacist who is offering the influenza immunisation is invited. So is the manager of the nursing home; he declines but sends a list of patients registered with the practice who have been immunised.
- The pharmacist pointing out that he cannot divulge the names of people he has immunised. He already gives people a card with a record of their immunisation. The nurse he employs will ask people to inform their own doctor that they have been immunised. A postscript is added to reminder letters asking people to notify the practice if they have received 'flu immunisation elsewhere.
- Slips of paper with spaces for recording name, address and date of birth of patient, together with the batch number of the vaccine are prepared and put with vaccines. All health staff who carry vaccine pledge to fill one in for each patient they immunise. The receptionist responsible for data entry will enter information from the recording slips.
- Notices being changed in the waiting room so that patients are encouraged to inform the practice if they have been immunised.
- Cards being kept at the reception desk to record details of all patients who tell the receptionists that they do not want immunisation or have had an immunisation elsewhere. The district nurses, practice nurses and doctors agree to record any patient who informs them they do not want immunisation, or has already had it, and let the responsible receptionist know.
- Completing Table 13.1.

Table 13.1:   Role and responsibilities checklist – *for each task tick the box for each team member who has a role or responsibility – then note your role and responsibilities for the task*

Completed by: _____

Task	Doctor	Practice nurse	District nurse	Reception team	Practice manager	Pharmacist	Other	What are your roles and your responsibilities?
			Primary care team member					
Identifying patients who should be included on the register	✔	✔	✔	✔	✔	✔	✔	*e.g. Making sure that people suspected, but not confirmed, of having the condition are **not** included on the register*
Identifying all those who have had influenza immunisation, those who should not have it and those who have declined	✔	✔	✔	✔	✔	✔	✔	*All members of the team need to participate to make this work well*
Task 3								
Task 4								
Task 5								

What extra resources might this require?

- Time for everyone involved to attend the practice meeting.
- The reminder letters about coming for a 'flu vaccination have to be altered to ask people to notify the practice if they have received immunisation elsewhere.
- Slips of paper with spaces for recording names, addresses and dates of birth of patients, together with the batch numbers of vaccine have to be printed, and time spent completing them.
- The practice secretary has to prepare new notices for the waiting room so that patients are encouraged to inform the practice if they have been immunised.
- Receptionists, district nurses, practice nurses and doctors have to make time to note down any patient who informs them that they do not want an influenza immunisation, or have had it elsewhere, and let the responsible receptionist know. She (or he) needs enough time to enter all the additional data.

The outcomes

These might include.

- A more complete record of those who have been immunised.
- Improved recording of those who have declined immunisation.
- A record of those who are excluded from the targets because of allergy or adverse reactions to influenza immunisation.

How would you demonstrate that you have achieved your outcomes?

- A search to establish the proportion of people on the practice list invited to have influenza immunisation, who have had it between September and March.
- Establishing the proportion of those invited who had not responded to three invitations or had declined immunisation and recording these as additional exclusions for this season.

(For a problem case example of smoking cessation advice see Chapter 10, page 139.)

Example problem case 2

Problem Case:

The practice receives a circular letter from the secondary care respiratory clinic, informing you that patients with COPD who are discharged from hospital will be issued with self-management plans to try to avoid further 'unnecessary admissions'. The letter says that an outreach specialist nurse will be supervising the implementation of this arrangement. You are asked 'to ensure that patients have sufficient medication' to be able to initiate antibiotic and steroid courses as directed by their self-management plans. The patients will also 'be required to attend six physiotherapy sessions' for rehabilitation.

Who do you need in your team?

You might want a team that includes:

Patients and carers
Practice nurses
GPs
Clerical staff
District nurses
Pharmacist
Practice manager
Physiotherapist
Specialist respiratory nurse.

Where you are now

The doctors and practice nurses agree that they do not know enough about self-management plans for COPD and are unclear how this will affect their own patient management and their workload. They deplore the imposition of this scheme without consultation and are angry about the implication that patients are admitted 'unnecessarily' to hospital.

What you do next

This might include.

- Asking any patients with COPD (or their carers) who have been recently discharged from hospital how they feel about their self-management plan.
- The GP and practice nurse who lead on COPD composing a letter to the responsible hospital specialist expressing their disappointment at the lack of consultation about these plans with a copy to their PCO. They ask if the specialist nurse can attend a practice or PCO area meeting to explain what is proposed and for more information about what the self-management plans involve.[2]
- The audit clerk extracting the names of patients on the COPD register who have been admitted to hospital in the last year. The GP and practice nurse who lead on COPD review the records for avoidable factors. They present their findings at a significant event meeting.
- At the significant event audit meeting, the team agreeing to review the medication of people on the COPD register for optimal management, including whether they are steroid responsive (and should have steroid rescue medication in reserve) and negotiating with patients if they wish to initiate antibiotic medication themselves at home. The reception staff are fully informed so that they can field any queries, or pass them on appropriately. The pharmacist is asked to ensure that any antibiotics and steroids that patients hold in reserve for emergencies have their expiry dates added to their labels; and in the case of liquid antibiotics are not 'made up' as they would then expire in 7 to 14 days.
- The practice inviting one of the physiotherapists running the rehabilitation scheme to come to talk at a lunchtime meeting. The local physiotherapists in the community clinic also attend and a useful exchange of views results.

What extra resources might this require?

- Only a few patients with COPD (or their carers) have recently been discharged from hospital with a self-management plan, so it is relatively easy for the GPs to ask for their feedback during an appointment that is booked at double the usual length.
- The GP and practice nurse who lead on COPD have to find time to compose the letter to the responsible hospital specialist and to read the information about self-management plans.
- The audit clerk needs designated time for performing the search for patients on the COPD register who have been admitted to hospital in the last year. The GP and practice nurse who lead on COPD have to set aside time to review the records, collating and presenting their findings at a significant event meeting.
- All staff need designated time for the significant event audit meeting. The practice secretary needs time to write up the account and action plan and to distribute them to all concerned.
- Time for a lunchtime meeting must be allocated and the practice manager or secretary have time to organise it.

The outcomes

These might include.

- Improved understanding of what self-management plans involve.
- Possibly improved management of COPD – but see the reference that suggested that research results are inconclusive.[2]
- Improved structured reviews of medication for patients with COPD.
- Improved relationships with the physiotherapy team.
- An extra resource (the specialist respiratory nurse) for patients with COPD, their carers and the clinical team.

How would you demonstrate that you have achieved your outcomes?

- Feedback from patients on the COPD register (and their carers) about how their condition is managed after 12 months.
- A report of medication reviews after 12 months.
- A significant event audit of a selected number of patient admissions for avoidable factors.

Problem case exercise

Problem Case:

One of the respiratory consultants in your area is sending patient letters to the practice categorising people as having 'COPD Stage 0'. Looking at the *Global Initiative for Chronic Obstructive Lung Disease*[3] the lead for COPD management finds that these patients do not fall into the category of COPD as defined under the guidelines for the GMS contract. This makes difficulties for the clerical staff who are responsible for adding people to the COPD register from discharge letters, and the practice is unsure how to manage this group of patients.

Who do you want in your team?

Where you are now

What you do next

Continued

What extra resources might this require?

The outcomes

How would you demonstrate that you have achieved your outcomes?

Why chronic obstructive pulmonary disease (COPD) is important

Chronic obstructive pulmonary disease is a major cause of death and disability.[4] In your PCO there are likely to be 54 to 55 deaths from COPD each year (compared with only two to three deaths per annum from asthma). Up to 25% of deaths from COPD occur before retirement age. By 2020, COPD is forecast to become the fifth most frequent cause of death.[5] In the UK, as many as one in eight medical admissions are due to COPD and in early January 2004 emergency admissions rose dramatically.[6]

The prevalence of COPD is greatest in socio-economically deprived people. The underlying cause is unknown and still under investigation. The genetic susceptibility to the disease is also being studied. Diagnosis is based on the history together with spirometry. The quality and outcomes framework guidance says that you should think about a diagnosis of COPD in any patient who has symptoms of persistent cough, sputum production or breathlessness and/or a history of exposure to risk factors to the disease.

The main risk factor for COPD is cigarette or other types of tobacco smoking. Other causes of COPD may include:

- occupational dust and chemicals (vapours, irritants and fumes) when prolonged or intense
- indoor air pollution from biomass fuel (wood, dung, etc.) used for cooking and heating in poorly ventilated dwellings
- outdoor air pollution, e.g. car fumes.

What is COPD?

COPD is a disease state characterised by airflow limitation that is not fully reversible. The airflow limitation is usually progressive and associated with an abnormal inflammatory response of the lungs to irritation. The symptoms are usually cough, production of sputum and breathlessness on exertion. Episodes of sudden worsening of the symptoms often occur. Other diagnostic labels included in COPD include:

- chronic bronchitis
- emphysema
- chronic obstructive airways disease
- chronic airways limitation
- some cases of chronic asthma.

Asthma shows reversible airflow limitation, although some chronic asthma may blur into COPD when the reversibility is not complete. Chronic bronchitis is defined as the presence of cough and sputum production for at least three months in each of two consecutive years, not necessarily with airflow limitation. Emphysema, defined as the destruction of the alveoli, is a pathological term but is often used loosely as a clinical diagnosis.

The criteria for the diagnosis of COPD under the GMS contract are that:

- the patient has a forced expiratory volume (FEV_1) of less than 70% of predicted normal (NICE[7] sets this at 80%)
- the patient has a FEV_1/FVC (forced vital capacity) ratio (that is, ratio of volume of air expired in one second to the total volume of air maximally expired) of less than 70%
- there is less than a 15% response on the reversibility test.

The guidelines from the *Global Initiative for Chronic Obstructive Lung Disease (GOLD)*[3] shown in Box 13.1 provide a useful tool for management.

Box 13.1:   Therapy guidelines from *GOLD* at each stage of COPD[3]

Stage	*Characteristics*	*Treatment options*
All		Avoidance of risk factors Influenza immunisation
Stage 0: At risk	Chronic symptoms Exposure to risk factors Normal spirometry	As above
Stage I: Mild	FEV_1/FVC less than 70% FEV_1 at or more than 80% with or without symptoms	Add short-acting bronchodilator when needed
Stage II: Moderate	FEV_1/FVC less than 70% FEV_1 between 50 and 80% with or without symptoms	Add regular treatment with one or more long-acting bronchodilators Add rehabilitation
Stage III: Severe	FEV_1/FVC less than 70% FEV_1 between 30 and 50% with or without symptoms	Add inhaled corticosteroids if has repeated exacerbations
Stage IV: Very severe	FEV_1/FVC less than 70% FEV_1 less than 30% with chronic respiratory failure or cor pulmonale	Add long-term oxygen if has respiratory failure. Consider surgical treatments, e.g. bullectomy or lung transplantation

What should you do, when and how?

You need access to spirometry testing. Spirometry uses a spirometer to measure how effectively and how quickly an individual can breathe out to empty the lungs. The curve measured is called the spirogram and measures volume against time. A booklet on spirometry can be downloaded from the British Thoracic Society website as well as several other useful information booklets on COPD.[8]

You might buy a spirometer if you don't already have one – or consider upgrading to one that downloads results automatically on to your computer software. If you are to carry out spirometry in your practice, staff must be trained and the equipment maintained and serviced. You might access a service funded by your PCO or use a lung function clinic in secondary care. Pharmaceutical companies may fund respiratory technicians or trained nurses to work in practices and can be a useful resource when the register is first being set up.

Setting it up

To start with, you will want to ensure that all patients with a new suspected diagnosis have this confirmed by spirometry. A suitably trained practice nurse or technician can do this. Then you might progress to reviewing all patients who:

- have regular or frequent oral steroids for respiratory distress
- are on anticholinergic medication
- have home oxygen (you may need to specifically ask for the lung function results from secondary care)
- are over 40 years of age, have a diagnosis of asthma and a history of smoking (you could start more slowly by selecting those over 50 years initially).

Continuation management of COPD

- Although the quality and outcomes framework only requires spirometry and checks on inhaler technique every two years as given in Table 13.2, it may be easier to set up an annual review combined with a medication review.
- Use the opportunity to discuss smoking cessation, as many patients with COPD are very resistant to suggestions that they should stop smoking despite their increasing disability.
- Decide who is going to do these checks – suitably trained nurses are often less threatening for patients and have better skills in this area than doctors. They might include in the review:
  - symptom assessment
  - checking frequency of repeat ordering of inhalers
  - smoking status and smoking cessation advice if required
  - inhaler use and technique (patients need a large volume spacer)
  - type of inhaler and whether newer breath-activated inhalers should be prescribed where older types are being used
  - spirometry
  - oxygen saturation with a finger probe pulse oximeter
  - advice about influenza immunisations if required
  - advice about pneumococcal immunisation
  - support and encouragement about diet, exercise and daily living activities.
- Develop a protocol for referral to secondary care. The guidance notes for the quality and outcomes framework suggest referral for patients with an FEV_1 of less than 50% who have disabling symptoms. Some areas have out-reach specialist nurses who can help patients with the management of their condition at home, once their diagnosis and treatment has been organised.[9]
- Have a mechanism for adding patients to the register when they have been diagnosed in secondary care.
- Invite all patients on the COPD register to have influenza immunisation. Make arrangements for those who are housebound.

What are the outcomes?

Maximise your outcome points by concentrating on the overlapping areas in different domains. For example, smoking and smoking cessation also appear in asthma, coronary heart disease, diabetes, hypertension and stroke. Checking inhaler technique and influenza immunisation also appears in the asthma outcomes and, for

Table 13.2: Quality and outcomes measures for COPD

Criteria	Maximum thresholds (minimum 25%) (%)	Points
The practice can produce a register of patients with COPD	Compatible with expected prevalence	5
A new diagnosis of COPD after 1 April 2003 has been confirmed by spirometry including reversibility testing	90	5
All patients on the COPD register have had the diagnosis confirmed by spirometry including reversibility testing	90	5
All patients on the COPD register have a record of their smoking status recorded in the last 15 months	90	6
Patients on the COPD register who smoke have a record that smoking cessation advice has been offered in the last 15 months	90	6
Patients on the COPD register have a record of their FEV_1 in the last 27 months	70	6
Patients on the COPD register using inhalers have a record that their inhaler technique has been checked in the last 2 years*	90	6
Patients on the COPD register have had influenza immunisation in the preceding September to March[†]	85	6

*Exception report patients on the COPD register who are not on inhalers.
[†]Failure to respond to three invitations for influenza immunisation or documented refusal can be exception coded each year. An adverse reaction or allergy can be exception coded permanently.

some patients, it will be difficult to decide into which category they fall. Where patients could be eligible for either register, the guidance for the quality indicators suggests that they are monitored on the asthma register.

Some of the information will come from secondary care when tests are carried out there, for example at a chest clinic. Set up procedures to record this information in the electronic medical record so that tests are not repeated unnecessarily and un-economically.

What are the challenges?

- The diagnoses of COPD and asthma overlap especially in older patients.
- Patients with COPD often minimise their disability and do not want to be diagnosed with a disabling condition.

- Spirometry has not been used in primary care until recently and there may be a large backlog of patients who require testing. After this backlog has been cleared, demand will flatten out and make investment in this area uneconomic.
- Many patients with disabling symptoms of COPD have other medical conditions.
- Resistance to smoking cessation is often considerable.
- Management is often not systematic because patients are seen when they have an exacerbation.

What can you do to make it more likely that you will succeed?

- Agree that one health professional (usually a practice nurse with extra training) will be responsible for monitoring the systematic care of patients with COPD.
- Involve patients and carers in the management of their condition, so that they understand the need for medical intervention and stopping smoking.
- Make sure every health professional has access to the guidelines for treating patients with COPD so that there is consistent management when exacerbations occur.
- Continue to manage the medical condition of those patients who are unable to stop smoking (without alienating them).
- Negotiate with your PCO to maximise spirometry testing opportunities initially without the need for massive investment of resources.

Further reading

Chambers R, Wakley G and Pullan A (2004) *Demonstrating Your Competence 4: respiratory disease, mental health, diabetes and dermatology*. Radcliffe Publishing, Oxford.

References

1 Department of Health (2004) *Update on the Influenza and Pneumococcal Immunisation Programmes*. Department of Health, London. www.dh.gov.uk/assetRoot/04/08/73/40/04087340.pdf

2 Monninkhof EM, van der Valk PDLPM, van der Palen J *et al.* (2004) Self-management education for chronic obstructive pulmonary disease (Cochrane Review). In: *The Cochrane Library, Issue 3*. John Wiley & Sons Ltd, Chichester.

3 *Global Initiative for Chronic Obstructive Lung Disease* available to download from www.brit-thoracic.org.uk/copd/consortium.html

4 Calverley PMA and Walker P (2003) Chronic obstructive pulmonary disease. *Lancet.* **362**: 1053–61.

5 Office for National Statistics (1999) *Mortality Statistics; Cause: England and Wales 1998*. Government Statistical Service, London.

6 Price D and Duerden M (2003) Chronic obstructive pulmonary disease (editorial). *BMJ.* **326**: 1046–7.

7 National Institute for Clinical Excellence (2004) *CG12 Chronic Obstructive Pulmonary Disease*: NICE guideline. www.nice.org.uk/Docref.asp?d=106421

8 www.brit-thoracic.org.uk/copd/consortium.html

9 Hermiz O, Comino E, Marks G *et al.* (2002) Randomised controlled trial of home based care of patients with chronic obstructive pulmonary disease. *BMJ.* **325**: 938–42.

14

Epilepsy

To explore how your primary care team might work together to improve the management of patients with epilepsy you can review a case (or cases) with which your team has been involved. You may prefer to use the two example cases at the start of this chapter. Read through them quickly before working on the problem case exercise (*see* page 200), or just photocopy Table 1.1 on page 7 to develop your own problem case. Include in your team people who will join in the problem-based learning discussion and be part of the solutions.

If you feel that you have insufficient knowledge to guide you in completing the problem-based learning, use the summary about epilepsy in the second part of this chapter and follow up the references if you need to learn more.

Example problem case 1

Problem Case:

When auditing the register for patients with epilepsy, it becomes obvious that a large number of patients with this diagnosis have not had a review for many years.

Who do you need in your team?

You might want a team that includes:

Patients
Clerical and secretarial staff – to code entries
GPs
Practice nurses.

Where you are now

Before panicking and recalling large numbers of people, ensure that entries on the epilepsy disease register are correct. The way in which the register of patients with epilepsy is compiled and maintained will affect how well you can demonstrate the quality outcomes.

What you do next

This might include checking how the search for setting up the disease register was conducted then:

- Taking off all patients with a diagnosis of epilepsy who are not on antiepileptic medication and keeping them on a separate list.
- A clinician, probably a GP, should go through the medical records of people on this list to see if the diagnosis of epilepsy has ever been confirmed. If not, modify the medical record to include the new diagnosis noting the reason for the alteration. If the diagnosis was confirmed in the past, then you could arrange a review to establish if any treatment is required to control seizures.
- Taking all patients off the epilepsy disease register who are on antiepileptic drugs for other indications, such as pain control.
- Adding to the disease register when letters including the diagnosis of epilepsy are received from secondary care.
- Arranging a regular pattern of reviews for patients remaining on the register, perhaps by linking this to their birthday month so that the process is spread out and easier for patients to remember.
- Being flexible in the way in which patients are reviewed. Someone who is employed and is seizure-free may prefer to answer review questions without physically attending the surgery. Allow them to give information about when they last had a seizure and whether they have any problems with their medication by telephone, email or letter.
- Ensuring that young people are entered on the disease register on their 16th birthday.
- Completing Table 14.1.

What extra resources might this require?

- Training for all staff who are responsible for coding and setting up patients' registers.
- Protected time for a clinician, probably one of the GPs, to go through the medical records of people on this list to see if the diagnosis has been confirmed.
- Protected time for correcting and maintaining the epilepsy register, including adding information about those managed in secondary care.
- Specified staff to organise the call and recall for a regular pattern of reviews for patients remaining on the register.
- Piloting the way in which patients are reviewed by including questions that you want answered in the call and recall notice and inviting patients to telephone or write in with information if they do not wish to attend. Asking patients for feedback about how they would like to participate. Offering other services at the same time such as a blood pressure and weight checks.

The outcomes

These might include.

- The epilepsy register only identifies those patients on antiepileptic medication.
- The register excludes those receiving antiepileptic drugs for other conditions.
- The register includes those diagnosed and managed in secondary care.
- Patients on the register are reviewed at least annually.

How would you demonstrate that you have achieved your outcomes?

- Audits of the epilepsy disease register show that those listed fall into the correct categories.
- Audits show that patients have a regular review at least annually.

Example problem case 2

Problem Case:

The register for patients with epilepsy has been compiled by searching for antiepileptic drugs and an automatic message added to the computerised repeat prescription for people to attend 'for a review of their epilepsy' when no more repeats are available. The GP reports at a practice meeting that he has had two angry patients this morning who complained that they have been stigmatised with a diagnosis of epilepsy. Both are taking antiepileptic drugs for chronic pain control.

Who do you need in your team?

You might want a team that includes:

Practice manager
Clerical and secretarial staff managing repeat prescriptions
Patients
GPs
Practice nurses.

Where you are now

The member of staff responsible for administration of the disease register has made a mistaken assumption that all patients on antiepileptic medication suffer from epilepsy.

What you do next

This might include.

- Apologising to the patients who complained and thanking them for drawing this to your attention, informing them about the action that will be taken.
- Immediately changing the wording of the message on the repeat prescription to invite patients for a review of their medication, with no mention of epilepsy.
- Revising the current criteria for inclusion on the epilepsy register so that it does not merely state 'being on anticonvulsant medication'.
- Reconsidering whether an automated message on a repeat prescription is the best way of involving patients in contributing to a dialogue with a health professional about their epilepsy.

Table 14.1: Role and responsibilities checklist – *for each task tick the box for each team member who has a role or responsibility – then note your role and responsibilities for the task*

Completed by: _____

| Task | Primary care team member | | | | | | | What are your roles and your responsibilities? |
	Doctor	Practice nurse	Clerical staff	Reception team	Practice manager	Practice secretary	Other	
Identifying patients who should be included on the register	✔	✔	✔	✔	✔	✔	✔	*e.g. Making sure that people suspected, but not confirmed, of having the condition are **not** included on the register*
Task 2								
Task 3								
Task 4								
Task 5								

- Go through repeat prescription requests to detect other examples to prevent other patients being falsely labelled as having epilepsy in an automated message.

What extra resources might this require?

- Look at the practice complaints procedure and see what needs to be done and by whom. If they are informal complaints, a letter from the GP and practice manager is appropriate.
- The staff member(s) responsible for messages on the repeat prescription must change the wording of the message.
- Make time for revision of the criteria for inclusion on the epilepsy register and for training for staff who are compiling the disease register.
- Ask for a volunteer, and find protected time, to contact a self-help society or invite patients to a meeting as to how you can best plan medication reviews in general. Feedback to the practice team so that a protocol can be drawn up.

The outcomes

These might include patients being reviewed appropriately and in ways that they find comfortable or convenient.

How would you demonstrate that you have achieved your outcomes?

- Outcomes of regular reviews of people on the epilepsy register can be substantiated.
- An increase in the number of people who are seizure-free can be demonstrated over a period of (say) three years.

Problem case exercise

Problem Case:

The practice receives a complaint after a young man with epilepsy was found dead in bed.[1] The young man had not been seen in the practice for about three years. The last hospital letter in his medical record states that he had been referred to the epilepsy specialist nurse, but that is dated several months ago. His record of medication does not confirm regular issues of antiepileptic medication and it is not clear whether he has been receiving other medication from secondary care.

Who do you need in your team?

Where you are now

What you do next

Continued

What extra resources might this require?

The outcomes

How would you demonstrate that you have achieved your outcomes?

Why epilepsy is important

Epilepsy is a common chronic neurological condition. Available data indicate an annual incidence of 40 to 70 per 100 000 population in developed countries, and a lifetime prevalence of five to ten per 1000.[2] Epilepsy is not a diagnosis but a symptom of an underlying neurological disorder with a wide range of causes. Although diagnosis of epilepsy can be straightforward, it can also be a difficult clinical challenge. Misdiagnosis is common and according to the literature the rate of misdiagnosis in the UK lies between 20 and 31%.[2] Human and financial costs of an incorrect diagnosis are considerable.

There are more than 350 000 people with epilepsy in the UK. The majority of people with epilepsy (80%) have total control of their symptoms with long-term drug treatment.[3]

What is epilepsy?

Abnormal electrical discharges in the brain cause fits (also called seizures), during which the affected person may temporarily lose consciousness. Epilepsy can start at any age, but children are more affected than adults. In about three-quarters of affected people, epilepsy develops before the age of 20 years. Children with epilepsy are usually managed by specialists in secondary care, but should be added to the practice disease register of patients with epilepsy from the age of 16 years.

A new diagnosis is based on a detailed account of the events immediately before, during and after the attack. Eye-witness accounts can be useful but can be obscured by faulty recollection and emotional distress. More than one attack is needed for a diagnosis. An electroencephalogram (EEG) can be diagnostic if carried out during an attack, but is often not specific enough for diagnosis. Sometimes people with true epilepsy have a normal EEG and those without epilepsy may show some abnormality. Imaging tests are not necessary for every patient with epilepsy. CT or MRI scans are usually reserved for people who developed epilepsy later in life. People with *primary* generalised seizures have normal scans and do not need imaging tests. Some people with partial seizures may need imaging depending on the age the epilepsy started, the type of fit and how well the epilepsy is controlled.

Seizures are classified into categories and this helps in the management for the initial choice of medication.[4] The two main categories are partial seizures either with or without impairment of consciousness, and generalised seizures of various types.

- **Simple partial seizures**: twitching, numbness, sweating, dizziness or nausea, a strong sense of déjà vu, and disturbances to hearing, vision, smell or taste.
- **Complex partial seizures**: plucking at clothes, smacking lips, swallowing repeatedly or wandering around. The person is not aware of their surroundings or of what they are doing.
- **Atonic seizures**: sudden loss of muscle control causes the person to fall to the ground. Recovery is quick.
- **Myoclonic seizures**: brief forceful jerks that can affect the whole body or just part of it. The jerking could be severe enough to make the person fall.
- **Absence seizures**: the person may appear to be daydreaming or switching off. They are momentarily unconscious and totally unaware of what is happening around them.

People with epilepsy can be grouped into:[5]

1   **Idiopathic (primary) epilepsy**: no obvious cause is found but where other family members are often affected. About 60% of people fall into this group.
2   **Cryptogenic epilepsy**: the cause is suspected but cannot be confirmed by tests.
3   **Symptomatic (secondary) epilepsy**: the cause is obvious such as following a head injury, meningitis, encephalitis, a brain tumour, or birth injury.

What should we do, when and how?

- Refer patients suspected of having epilepsy to a neurologist or paediatrician with expertise in neurology. Patients should be seen within four weeks of referral.[4]
- If a patient has focal neurological signs, severe prolonged or frequent seizures admit him/her to secondary care or discuss their management with the specialist.[4]
- Give information to the patient, relatives and carers about what to do during a seizure.
  - Remove the person from harm (e.g. proximity to a fire).
  - Do not put anything in the patient's mouth.
  - Put the person in the recovery position as soon as possible – if the seizure (convulsion) lasts more than five minutes, call for paramedics to come via the ambulance service.
  - Stay with the person after the seizure for at least 20 minutes and reassure them.
  - Tuck the person up in bed to sleep it off as soon as possible – while the individual is asleep, check him or her at intervals to ensure that the seizure has not started again.
- Give general information to the patients, relatives and carers about epilepsy and sources for more support and information.[6] Give advice about employment issues[6] and driving regulations.[7]
- A specialist usually starts drug treatment and you should prescribe by brand as not all preparations are bio-equivalent. Include in your monitoring.[4]
  - Ensure that the patient fully understands the importance of taking the medication exactly as prescribed – concordance works better than compliance
  - Seizures, side-effects, or the introduction of medication that may affect the metabolism of the antiepileptic drug, should prompt a review or measurement of serum levels
  - Measure serum levels of phenytoin but alter dosages only if required by the clinical picture – there is no evidence to support routine monitoring of other antiepileptic drugs.
- Refer patients where seizure control is inadequate, or when there is a specific issue such as pregnancy.[8,9]
- Treatment should be tailored to the patient and type of seizures occurring. If treatment is not controlling the seizures refer back for further expert advice.[10,11]

What are the outcomes?

The ideal outcomes for people with epilepsy is for them to be seizure free, with no side-effects from their medication and leading a normal lifestyle. This is achievable for the majority of patients with epilepsy. However, about 20% of patients develop refractory epilepsy and it is this group who present a challenge to healthcare professionals to optimise their quality of life. A good service in primary care to patients with epilepsy would be the practice team being able to demonstrate:

- a database of all patients with epilepsy
- periodic review of patients with intractable epilepsy
- periodic review of patients on older antiepileptic drugs, e.g. annually
- members of the primary care team with particular expertise in the management of patients with epilepsy, e.g. a practice nurse and/or a GP
- close links with the local epilepsy liaison nurse and neurosciences services

- sources of information for healthcare professionals and patients (written and on-line).[6]

Quality measures in epilepsy

For many practices this is a new area to demonstrate their quality of care. Although this is not a high-scoring domain, the four indicators will show that you are improving the care of patients with epilepsy and reducing seizure frequency (*see* Table 14.2).

Table 14.2:   Quality and outcomes measures for epilepsy

Criteria	Maximum thresholds (minimum 25%) (%)	Points
A register of patients receiving drug treatment for epilepsy	Practice prevalence in line with national/local prevalence figures	2
Patients over 16 years of age on drug treatment have a seizure frequency recorded in the last 15 months	90	4
Patients over 16 years of age on drug treatment have had a medication review in the last 15 months	90	4
Patients over 16 years of age on drug treatment have a record that they have been seizure-free for 12 months	70	6

Gaining points in this clinical domain will also contribute towards your quality outcomes in holistic care. Most GP software systems have a template for recording the management of epilepsy. You should record the following.

- Seizure type and frequency, including date of last seizure.
- Antiepileptic drug therapy, ensuring prescribing by brand, and dosage.
- Any side-effects from medication.
- The management plan for the coming year.
- Any other issues such as contraception, driving or employment.

Check that the epilepsy disease register only includes those patients with a confirmed diagnosis of epilepsy, not those taking antiepileptic medication for pain control (*see* Problem case example 2 on page 197). A designated member of the practice team should have responsibility for recalling those patients who need an annual review on a rolling programme. Currently there is no Read code for recording freedom from seizures, so you may need to allocate a practice code so that audits can easily retrieve all the information you require. You might exclude patients from the fourth indicator if they are on maximum tolerated medication but still have poor control, e.g. with severe brain damage, or patients who have unacceptable side-effects with medication.

What are the challenges?

- Most practices are not providing structured care.
- Patients with epilepsy are unused to medical interest in their condition and often prefer to remain hidden because of perceived or actual prejudice.
- There are insufficient secondary care specialists so that recommended waiting times for referral for diagnosis may be exceeded.
- Regular review will increase the number of patients who need specialist advice to improve their outcomes – further increasing waiting times for neurology opinions.
- Practice team members having generally poor knowledge of the management of epilepsy in primary care.
- There are insufficient numbers of specialist liaison nurses for epilepsy so that promised support for newly diagnosed or patients with difficult to manage epilepsy is not forthcoming.

What can you do to make it more likely that you will succeed?

- Arrange in-house training for the practice team so that it is more confident in managing less severe problems.
- Arrange in-house or voluntary organisation-assisted education for patients, carers, relatives and staff.
- Feedback on deficiencies in specialist care and specialist liaison nurses to your PCO.
- Consider with the PCO if there is a place for a service provided by practitioners with a special interest (PwSI) and who would train to provide this.[12]

References

1   British Epilepsy Association. *Sudden Unexpected Death in Epilepsy*. www.epilepsy.org.uk/info/sudep.html

2   National Institute of Clinical Excellence (2003) *Costs of Epilepsy Misdiagnosis*. www.nice.org.uk/pdf/APPENDIX_G_Costs_of_epilepsy_misdiagnosis.pdf

3   Scottish Intercollegiate Guidance Network (1997) *Diagnosis and Management of Epilepsy in Adults*. www.sign.ac.uk/pdf/qrg21.pdf

4   Epilepsy Action. *Principles of Epilepsy Management*. In: Foord-Kelcey (2004) *Guidelines*. **23**: 115–57. www.eguidelines.co.uk

5   British Brain and Spine Foundation (1999) *Epilepsy: a guide for patients and carers*. www.brainandspine.org.uk/pdf/epilepsy.pdf

6   www.epilepsy.org.uk

7   UK Driving Licence Regulations for Neurological Conditions. www.dvla.gov.uk/at_a_glance/ch1_neurological.htm

8   NICE (2004) *Guidelines on Management of Epilepsy*. www.nice.org.uk

9   Scottish Intercollegiate Guidance Network (1997) *The Management of Pregnancy in Women with Epilepsy*. www.sign.ac.uk/guidelines/sogap/sogap1.html

10   Feely M (1999) Drug treatment of epilepsy. *BMJ.* **318**: 106–9. http://bmj.bmjjournals.
     com/cgi/reprint/318/7176/106

11   Wakley G, Chambers R and Ellis S (2004) *Demonstrating Your Competence 3: cardiovascular
     and neurological conditions.* Radcliffe Publishing, Oxford. www.radcliffe-oxford.com

12   www.gpwsi.org

15

Cancer and palliative care

Most patients who eventually receive a diagnosis of cancer initially present to a primary care clinician. A person with cancer spends almost all of their time living at home. Most express the wish to die there, although less than 30% actually do. Active management of cancer does occur in the secondary care setting.[1] The role of primary care is extraordinarily important for a person with cancer, and their family. The primary care team is involved in every aspect of what has become widely known as the 'cancer journey'. This can be seen from the brief list that follows.

Cancer prevention

- New patient checks (opportunity to take and record a brief cancer family history).
- Healthy living – smoking cessation, healthy eating and the 'five a day' campaign of encouraging people to eat at least five pieces of fruit or vegetables per day.
- Providing encouragement for patients to attend screening and be aware of changes in their own bodies that might be significant.

Cancer screening

Getting the cervical smear programme right (in terms of quality assurance, training and access).

Cancer referral

- Being aware of the warning symptoms that might indicate malignant disease.
- Using the 14-day referral pathways appropriately.

Support after diagnosis

- Recognising physical, psychological and social implications of a cancer diagnosis.
- Being aware of the complications of outpatient treatment of cancers that may present to primary care and dealing with these appropriately.

Support for those who are not going to be cured

- Recognising and supporting patients who are living with their cancer rather than actively dying from it. (The increasing numbers of people in this group are possibly the biggest change in community cancer care in the last 20 years.)
- Recognising and supporting patients and their families as the illness reaches a terminal stage.

End of life care

- Planning for the more likely situations which occur during the terminal stages so that they do not become a crisis.
- Support for families and relatives following bereavement.

No individual member of a primary care team can do this on their own. Many of these tasks require skilled individuals performing well together if they are to be undertaken successfully. Palliative care is a particularly complex area for a primary care team. The situation can change very quickly and a perfectly sensible plan at 10 am can look inadequate or wrong at 4 pm the same day. Excellent communication within the team and with the patient and carers is fundamental.

Problem-based learning in cancer care

To explore how your primary care team might work together to improve the management of patients with cancer you can review a case (or cases) with which your team has been involved. You may prefer to use the three example cases at the start of this chapter. Read through them quickly before working on the problem case exercise (*see* page 215), or just photocopy Table 1.1 on page 7 to develop your own problem case. Include in your team people who will join in the problem-based learning discussion and be part of the solutions.

If you feel that you have insufficient knowledge to guide you in completing the problem-based learning, use the summary about cancer in the second part of this chapter and follow up the references if you need to learn more.

Example problem case 1

Problem Case:

Mrs Lump is a 38-year-old nursery nurse with a seven-year-old child. She was referred to the breast clinic by a GP locum working at the practice and has subsequently had a positive biopsy. Mrs Lump telephones the reception team in a distressed state.

Who do you need in your team?

You might want a team that includes:

Patient
Receptionists
GPs
Practice nurses
CPN or counsellor.

Where you are now

Consider the issues that might be important.

- Did the locum use the 14-day referral pathway?
- Did the patient have enough information after the consultation?
- Access to clinicians in the practice.
- How do the reception team/other staff deal with distressed patients?
- Can the practice handle these situations well every time?

What you do next

This might include.

- Producing a locum pack including referral pathway information.
- Reminding everyone about the current 14-day guidelines and pathways for local services.
- Arranging some role play training for staff so that patients who are obviously distressed are dealt with appropriately.
- Completing Table 15.1.

What extra resources might this require?

- The practice secretary and the GPs need time to produce a locum pack.
- The guidelines and pathways could be added to a desktop pack either in a folder or on the computer – but someone will need time to do it.
- Protected time in an educational session could be allocated to a CPN or counsellor to run a session on how to manage acutely distressed patients.

The outcomes

These might include.

- All the practice team, including any locum, knowing about guidelines and pathways for suspected cancer.
- The practice team being better equipped to manage acutely distressed patients.

How would you demonstrate that you have achieved your outcomes?

- An audit shows that referrals are being channelled appropriately.
- Feedback confirms patients' appreciation of the skills and attitudes of the practice team.

Table 15.1: Role and responsibilities checklist – *for each task tick the box for each team member who has a role or responsibility – then note your role and responsibilities for the task*

Completed by: _____

Task	Primary care team member							What are your roles and your responsibilities?
	Doctor	*Practice nurse*	*District nurse*	*Receptionist*	*Counsellor*	*CPN*	*Other*	
Identifying patients who might have cancer								
Using the 14-day referral pathway								
Recording a cancer diagnosis within the practice								
Managing the complications of treatment for malignancy								
Task 5								
Task 6								

Example problem case 2

Problem Case:

Mrs Chest (a single parent with two children) comes to the surgery after her consultation with the surgical team at the hospital following a referral for a lump in her left breast. A faxed report detailing the confirmed malignant status of the lump is received by the practice an hour before she arrives.

Who do you need in your team?

You might want a team that includes:

Patients
Clerical and secretarial staff coding entries
GPs
Practice nurses.

Where you are now

How does information in an important fax get passed on to the doctor who is going to see the patient, as well as the doctor to whom the document is addressed? If there is important diagnostic data on this fax how, when and by whom will it be coded?

Who else within the team needs to know about Mrs Chest's diagnosis? How are they going to find out?

- A single parent with children is particularly vulnerable – consider the needs of the children. What does Mrs Chest want to say to them, does she want to say something to the school – does she need help?
- Within the bounds of confidentiality, do you as a team have a right to share clinical information with a school nurse or a local health visitor who may have contact with the children?

What you do next

This might include.

- Designing a policy for passing on urgent information within the practice.
- Reviewing data coding.
  - Add practice Read code for breast cancer (*see* page 218 for a list of codes along with suggestions for implementing them).
  - Add specific code 8BAV for 'cancer care review' to indicate that you have discussed the cancer diagnosis (this is a particular requirement of the QOF and it will be much easier for the team later if this code is entered now). If your practice does not use the computer system, ensure that Mrs Chest's name is appended to the cancer disease register along with a note that you have had a discussion with her about the diagnosis.

What extra resources might this require?

- The practice manager needs time to put in place procedures to manage faxes.
- Time for staff to discuss and become familiar with these procedures.
- Time for training on relevant codes for breast cancer and cancer review.

The outcomes

These might include.

- Urgent information passed on to the appropriate people.
- Coding of cancer and cancer reviews being done correctly and entries on to cancer registers completed.

How would you demonstrate that you have achieved your outcomes?

Review of a sample of medical records.

Problem Case continued:

Mrs Chest subsequently has an extended lumpectomy and is offered adjuvant chemotherapy.

Three days after her second cycle has been administered she develops a sore throat.

Who do you need in your team?

You might want a team that includes:

Patients
Receptionists managing appointment systems
Practice manager drawing up procedures
GPs
Practice nurses or nurse practitioners.

Where you are now

- Sore throats are often dealt with by telephone but the patient needs to know that this is not appropriate in this situation.
- The risk is neutropenic sepsis – how will the practice team be alerted to the possibility that this sore throat could be a sign of a potentially life-threatening condition?
- Should someone having chemotherapy sit in a busy waiting room?
- What are the local guidelines for using paracetamol with fever in someone having intensive chemotherapy?

What you do next

This might include.

- Using the practice computer system or a sticker on the notes to identify patients who may be immuno-compromised.
- Agreeing a policy concerning communication with patients who are on a 'high priority' list because of their recent diagnosis or potentially complex unstable healthcare needs.
- Checking with the local oncology unit for their guidelines for managing neutropenia. Almost all units will have a handout that they give to patients and many will have a primary care information sheet too.

What extra resources might this require?

- A designated person needs to flag the medical records of anyone who is immuno-compromised. There will not be many and a practice secretary could be trained to pick out the criteria from hospital letters.
- The practice team need time to discuss the management of sore throat queries and when further advice should be sought.
- A separate room should be available at the practice premises for anyone who requires 'quarantine' either for their protection or for the protection of others.

The outcomes

The potential risk of a sore throat complaint in immuno-compromised patients is recognised.

How would you demonstrate that you have achieved your outcomes?

Significant event review promotes reflective learning. The GMS contract allocates four quality points for having undertaken 12 such reviews in the preceding three years. Newly diagnosed cancer or palliative care cases with a home 'terminal care' component, are particularly identified as being appropriate.

Example problem case 3

Problem Case:

Mr Ping is a 66-year-old man known to have carcinoma of the prostate. His last prostate specific antigen (PSA) test was raised despite his regular goserelin injections. His wife contacts the practice and asks to speak to his GP because she is concerned about the increasing discomfort he is getting in his back.

Who do you need in your team?

You might want a team that includes:

Patient
Carer
Receptionists taking telephone calls
Practice manager drawing up procedures
GPs
Practice nurses or nurse practitioners.

Where you are now

Look at his last review by the practice or by secondary care to establish if this is a new problem, or one already under investigation or management. Look at how telephone contact is managed – when will the GP speak to his wife, can anyone else help until the GP is able to contact her, and should his wife be asked to ring back at a time when the GP can reasonably be expected to talk to her? The GP needs permission from the patient to talk to his wife about his medical condition, so may have to ask the wife to arrange an early review, rather than discussing this over the phone.

What you do next

This might include.

- Reviewing medical records to check if, and how often, you have recorded consent to discuss the medical condition with a named carer or carers.
- Asking patients and carers for feedback on the accessibility of telephone advice and contact with the practice team.
- GP review of the complaint of back pain in someone with a diagnosis of cancer. Look at how you distinguish between backache from common causes and that due to secondary deposits and at what stage you would want to discuss the case with the oncology team in order that they (or you, if your local referral arrangements allow) can arrange a scan.
- Selecting a few medical records of people on the cancer register to determine if the review consultation is thorough enough to pick up (minor) complaints like backache.
- Arranging a clinical practice meeting to discuss the findings of your record reviews and planning any action needed.
- Arranging an administrative practice meeting to discuss patient and carer feedback about telephone contact and planning any changes required.

What are the resources you need to achieve this?

- Time for a GP or a trained deputy to review medical records.
- Time for the practice manager or deputy to arrange for patient and carer feedback about telephone contact.
- Time for meetings about the results and for necessary changes.
- Maybe allocate more telephone contact time for GPs and nurses in the working day.

The outcomes

These might include.

- Improved telephone contact arrangements for patients and carers.
- Improved awareness of the significance and proper management of back pain in patients on the cancer register.
- Improved recording of consent to pass on information about the patient to others.

How would you demonstrate that you have achieved your outcomes?

- Repeat feedback about telephone contact.
- Repeat medical record reviews.

Problem case exercise

This is a continuation of Problem case example 3.

Problem Case continued:

Mr Ping has had radiotherapy for his lumbar vertebral metastasis (which didn't show up on a lumbar spine X-ray). He has had a good summer but has become increasingly emaciated and is now bed bound. His wife calls in to say that he is so weak he has not been able to take a drink for the last 24 hours and she is worried he will get dehydrated.

Who do you need in your team?

Where you are now

Continued

What you do next

What extra resources might this require?

The outcomes

How would you demonstrate that you have achieved your outcomes?

Why cancer diagnosis and management are important

More than one in three people in England will develop cancer at some stage in their lives. One in four will die of cancer. This means that, every year, over 200 000 people are diagnosed with cancer and around 120 000 people die from cancer.[2] These bald facts do not tell the whole story. Patients are living longer with their cancers than before. The average primary care team will have many more patients who are living with their cancers than previously.

A cancer diagnosis is still understandably feared by patients and their families. Aggressive treatment is debilitating and can seem overwhelming. The cancer journey can be thought of as a macabre big dipper ride, with moments of high elation interspersed with heart stopping sudden lows and persistent anxiety. The primary care team will make this as comfortable as possible.

What is included in the cancer register?

A cancer register is a complete list of patients within a practice who have been diagnosed as having malignant illness. It is difficult to compile this from historical Read codes because:

- The Read 'B' hierarchy includes a scattering of non-malignant and pre-malignant diagnoses throughout its structure, making a search on B type codes unrewarding. It can be done iteratively, i.e. by searching for the whole of the B chapter, noting codes that get thrown up for non-malignant conditions and adding them to a search as exclusions.
- Inexperienced coders often wrongly code malignancy as *cancer in situ* – so beware historical codes for these. Did the patient really have cancer *in situ* or a more significant illness?
- Sometimes cancers are coded via a histological diagnosis rather than a disease code – there is no way to know other than by looking – 'adenocarcinoma' can be coded like this rather than by organ system.
- Sometimes cancers are coded by operation rather than disease – e.g. 'AP resection' instead of 'malignant neoplasm of rectum'. Whilst a practice team that makes extensive use of a computer system would want to have both Read codes, there is no easy way of finding the disease from the surgical code without a great deal of clinical involvement.

Coding a new diagnosis

The current trend is to move away from Read code formularies to use the most appropriate clinical code for the condition instead. Unfortunately, search systems and QOF monitoring systems are not so sophisticated and look for defined Read subsets. If a practice has not developed a more sophisticated system for itself the simple code list from the original GMS contract support documentation is a good start.[1] Consider how you are going to limit yourselves to this pick list (*see* Box 15.1) as a practice. This will depend upon which clinical system you adopt but could be done by setting these up as preferred codes or as a template.

Box 15.1: Cancer diagnosis Read code pick list

Malig. Neoplasm Lip, Oral, Pharynx	B0zz.
Malig. Neoplasm Oesophagus	B10z.
Malig. Neoplasm Stomach	B11z.
Malig. Neoplasm Small Intestine	B12z.
Malig. Neoplasm Colon	B13..
Malig. Neoplasm Rectum	B141.
Malig. Neoplasm Liver	B152.
Malig. Neoplasm Gall Bladder	B160.
Malig. Neoplasm Pancreas	B17z.
Malig. Neoplasm Larynx	B21z.
Malig. Neoplasm Trachea NOS	B220z
Mesothelioma	B226.
Malig. Neoplasm Bronchus/Lung NOS	B22z.
Malig. Neoplasm Bone	B30z.
Ca Connective Tissue (e.g. sarcoma)	B31..
Malig. Melanoma Skin	B32
Malig. Neoplasm Female Breast	B34
Malig. Neoplasm Uterus (part unspecified)	B40..
Malig. Neoplasm Cervix Uteri	B41z.
Malig. Neoplasm Body of Uterus	B43..
Malig. Neoplasm Ovary	B440.
Malig. Neoplasm Vulva	B454.
Malig. Neoplasm Prostate	B46.
Malig. Neoplasm Testes	B47z.
Malig. Neoplasm Penis	B483.
Malig. Neoplasm Bladder	B49z.
Malig. Neoplasm Kidney	B4A..
Malig. Neoplasm Brain	B51..
Malig. Neoplasm Thyroid Gland	B53..
Malig. Neoplasm Lymph/Haemo Tiss	B6...
Hodgkin's Disease	B61..
Non-Hodgkin's Lymphoma	B627.
Multiple Myeloma	B630.
Acute Lymphoid Leukaemia	B640.
Chronic Lymphoid Leukaemia	B641.
Acute Myeloid Leukaemia	B650.
Chronic Myeloid Leukaemia	B651.

Putting it together

Identify all letters coming into the practice which discuss a cancer diagnosis.

- Mark these letters – perhaps with a highlighter letter 'C'.
- 'C' coded letters are passed to a staff member to cross-check that the diagnosis has been recorded on the computer system and been assigned a code from the pick list. If not, someone from the clinical team should add an appropriate code.

- The team member adds code 8BAV to confirm that a 'cancer care review' discussion has taken place in the practice, with the appropriate date. If there is no recorded discussion then an alert can be set up on the record or entered into the written notes.

What should you do, when and how?

Reviewing patients with a diagnosis of cancer

The GMS contract requires a review of cancer patients within six months of diagnosis. Whilst inserting the appropriate Read code will trigger QOF points it is not, in itself, a record of the needs of the patient and their family. Almost all patients diagnosed with cancer will contact the practice within six months of diagnosis. Some practices may have a policy for visiting or telephoning patients soon after a diagnosis of cancer has been made. Good communication skills are needed for these consultations. As they can be stressful for the health professional too, a simple checklist can be constructed and used as a paper aide mémoire. This same checklist could be converted into a computer template for ease of subsequent data recording as in Box 15.2.

Box 15.2:   Checklist for reviewing care needs in cancer cases

- Patient's understanding of condition and treatment
- Carer's understanding of condition and treatment and level of consent for sharing of information
- Understanding of what the hospital oncology team is doing
- Pathways to getting more information – local information centre, BACUP, Macmillan team
- Pathways to getting help – out-of-hours contacts, district nursing contacts, Macmillan team
- Benefits – sickness certification, DS1500 when appropriate, other benefits – may need welfare benefits help
- Involving other professionals – school nurses for families with school age children, health visitors for those with younger families

---

What are the outcomes?

The quality and outcomes framework on cancer management section is quite short (*see* Table 15.2).

Table 15.2:   Quality and outcomes measures for cancer

Criteria	Maximum thresholds (minimum 25%) (%)	Points
The practice can produce a register of all cancer patients diagnosed after 1 April 2003	In line with that expected	6
The percentage of patients with cancer diagnosed from 1 April 2003 with a review by the practice recorded within 6 months of confirmed diagnosis. This should include an assessment of support needs, if any, and a review of co-ordination arrangements with secondary care	90	6

What are the challenges?

The challenges of prevention, screening and diagnosis are no different to managing any other chronic disease. Earlier stages of cancer management require good organisation, a repertoire of health promotion strategies, and knowledge of disease processes and referral pathways. Once a cancer diagnosis has been made there are some specific challenges.

- Ability to deal with distress (good communication and consultation skills).
- Team organisation to deal with a patient dying at home.[3,4]
- Confidence to deal with increasingly complex problems if the patient develops more advanced illness.

What can you do to make it more likely that you will succeed?

You should review the resources you have within your team to deal with these challenges. Some members of the team will have better skills and confidence than others.

Ability to deal with distress (good communication and consultation skills)

Most of us feel uncomfortable about breaking bad news, or dealing with the 'fall out' from bad news delivered badly. Communication skills can be learned and improved with practice. Having a framework in mind helps you through these difficult consultations as shown in Box 15.3.

Box 15.3:   Dealing with distress: using the example of Mrs Chest (Problem case example 2)

A response to the initial distress might be.

Straightaway

- acknowledge her distress (be empathic)
- allow her to ventilate whatever emotion she has
- attempt to understand her current disease understanding (in terms of ideas, concerns, and expectations)
- decide about whether or not she is in a position to assimilate further information at all.

If Mrs Chest is not able to assimilate further information then you need to be quite directive.

- Check that she is safe or at least has a safety net of family and friends – encourage her to 'use them' for a while.
- Arrange to see her again – perhaps later that day, with her partner or a friend.
- Augment her safety net – with breast care nurses or Macmillan nurses (who are increasingly becoming cancer specialist care nurses rather than palliative care nurses. Local people may not be aware of this and mention of Macmillan can amplify anxiety if the role is not explained exactly), BACUP information or locally available help lines.

If Mrs Chest can assimilate further information, begin to align where 'she thinks she is' with where 'you think she is'. This will not be completely achieved at this consultation; you might not know enough facts to challenge any of her current beliefs. Be realistically optimistic without being untruthful (this is the true heart of a consultation with a person who has just had a serious diagnosis). You tend to want to be falsely optimistic – in a situation where you may have very little idea of the real status of the disease. If you are untruthful at this stage [*for example, saying 'these cancers are all curable you know…'; and the patient is subsequently shown to have metastatic spread*] you risk destroying the trust in your relationship with the patient – at the very time when she needs it most. On the other hand be aware that a person assimilates bad news in chunks and needs time to digest the news. Being honest does not mean that you have to tell a patient everything in one go, or to necessarily share your fears about their situation at this consultation.

And in conclusion
Conclude the consultation by offering further follow up with another team member or by arranging a further appointment.

Team organisation required to deal with a patient dying at home

This involves the whole team. Reception and administrative staff should be able to recognise such patients and families so that information can be 'fast tracked' to the relevant doctor or nurse. Prescriptions have to be provided quickly – often computer repeat lists become out of date within hours or days but leaving a request to be sorted at the bottom of a prescription query pile is disastrous. Know which of the local pharmacists is likely to have stocks of palliative care medication (midazolam and larger quantities of diamorphine can be particularly problematic). The medication and instructions for its use have to be in the house before the crisis! Contact the out-of-hours nursing and medical team about patients who are terminally ill. Use a transfer form (*see* Appendix 1). Some practices might prefer a standard or customised computer note summary instead of hand-completing the form.

Dealing with complex problems in advanced illness

This final section is mainly for clinical practitioners. We include it as Appendix 2 as it is a specialised field that is not relevant to the wider primary care team.

Further reading

Baile W and Buckman R (2000) SPIKES – a six-step protocol for delivering bad news: application to the patient with cancer. *The Oncologist.* **5(4)**: 302–11. http://theoncologist. alphamedpress.org

Faulkner A (1998) ABC of palliative care: communication with patients, families, and other professionals. *BMJ.* **316**: 130–2. http://bmj.bmjjournals.com/

The NHS Cancer Plan www.dh.gov.uk/assetRoot/04/01/45/13/04014513.pdf (or by typing 'NHS cancer plan' into www.google.co.uk)

The NHS Information Agency is developing a data set of codes which could be used as the basis for a practice designed template. www.nhsia.nhs.uk/cancer/pages/dataset/docs/Primary_care_dataset.pdf

The Primary Care Good Practice Guide – is a compilation of ideas from the primary care cancer collaborative. www.macmillan.org.uk/healthprofessionals/disppage.asp?id=2065

Useful information about the *Gold Standards framework* downloadable from the Macmillan Site www.macmillan.org.uk/healthprofessionals/disppage.asp?id=6875

Useful information about the *Liverpool Care Pathway for the dying patient* can be found at www.lcp-mariecurie.org.uk/ – examples of the pathway can be downloaded in pdf.

References

1   General Practitioners Committee/The NHS Confederation (2003) *Supporting Documentation for New GMS Contract.* British Medical Association, London.

2   Department of Health (2000) *The NHS Cancer Plan.* Department of Health, London.

3   Thomas K (2003) *Caring for the Dying at Home.* Radcliffe Medical Press, Oxford.

4   Ellershaw J (2003) *Care of the Dying – a pathway to excellence.* Oxford University Press, Oxford.

16

Patient safety in your practice

To explore how your primary care team might work together to improve patient safety in your practice you can review a case (or cases) with which your team has been involved. You may prefer to use the two example cases at the start of this chapter. Read through them quickly before working on the problem case exercise (see page 228), or photocopy Table 1.1 on page 7 and develop your own problem case with incidents from your own practice. This process of working together leads to better risk assessment, a deeper insight into potential problems and more effective solutions. Include in your team people who will join in the problem-based learning discussion and be part of the solutions.

If you feel that you have insufficient knowledge to guide you in completing the problem-based learning, use the summary about patient safety in the second part of this chapter and follow up the references if you need to learn more.

Example problem case 1

> **Problem Case:**
>
> During a busy morning surgery a GP pops into the back office to ask a receptionist to take a letter concerning a patient along to his consulting room, then answers a phone call whilst he is in the office. He had left the patient lying on the examination couch in the consulting room with the curtains drawn round with her two-year-old child playing on the floor. As the child shakes a bright yellow tub containing used sharps, her mother hears what she takes to be 'lego' bricks rattling inside. The receptionist enters the room just as the child is trying to open the red lid of the sharps container ... .

Who do you need in your team?

You might want a team that includes:

Reception staff
Practice manager
GP
Patients

Practice nurses
Healthcare assistants
Cleaners.

Where you are now

A serious injury has narrowly been avoided as the sharps container was in reach of a small child. The practice needs to identify:

- how this happened
- if its practice policy is flawed to allow such an incident
- what needs to be done to tighten up the system for handling sharps in the practice to prevent this happening again.

What you do next

This might include.

- The receptionist taking the container away from the child and placing it on top of the treatment trolley in the corner of the room out of the child's reach. She informs the GP about the incident and her action.
- The receptionist also reporting the incident to the practice manager.
- The practice manager arranging a risk assessment of all consultation and treatment rooms that day. An investigation discovers that the new cleaner had been giving that consultation room a thorough clean and had put the sharps container back on a lower shelf of the treatment trolley.
- The practice secretary being asked to produce notices for the patient notice board to ask parents, wherever possible, to bring or arrange for someone to look after their child, if the parent or carer needs to attend the surgery for a consultation, investigation or treatment.
- Sending an email to all GPs, nurses and healthcare assistants reminding them of the practice policy relating to the handling and disposal of sharps and of the need to remain vigilant when children are in the consultation/treatment areas.
- Using the incident as the focus of a significant event analysis exercise where the whole practice team identifies what went wrong and discusses what improvements it can make to prevent the situation happening again. The team agrees the following actions.
  - The practice manager will arrange for cleaners to have a formal induction training session on all health and safety practices including waste management, sharps handling and disposal and cross infection.
  - Healthcare assistants will check the sharps containers each morning when they restock the treatment/consultation rooms.
- Completing Table 16.1.

What extra resources might this require?

- The practice secretary needs time and resources to make posters for the waiting room.
- Patients and carers with small children will need to find other people to care for their children when attending for consultations.

- The practice manager needs time and the knowledge to investigate the incident, give an induction session to the cleaners and produce suitable written material to give to the cleaners to reinforce the messages.
- Cleaners need paid time to attend the induction session.
- Healthcare assistants need time to check each room. This may have to start earlier before others have started work, or stay on after people have finished in the evening. Their hours of employment may need adjusting, or more people be employed or other members of staff trained, to ensure that the task is performed consistently, even when people are away on holiday or taking sick leave.

The outcomes

These might include.

- A safer environment for patients, their children and for staff.
- Conditions for consultations for parents and carers with small children are more favourable.
- Other areas of risk may be identified at an early stage following the practice significant event meeting that raised participants' level of awareness of potential risks.

How would you demonstrate that you have achieved your outcomes?

The healthcare assistant's report to the practice manager that sharps boxes are always placed in a suitable position to avoid young children being able to pick them up.

Example problem case 2

Problem Case:

Dr Holiday had just returned from leave to full surgeries and a backlog of paperwork. Mrs Lower asked to be examined. Her cervical polyp had been removed three weeks ago but she was still getting a lot of smelly discharge. Dr Holiday picked up the bag containing the sterilised speculum, tore it open – and then noticed that it was cut open neatly at the other end. Looking more closely, there was a small amount of debris on the inside of the speculum. Hastily she found another for the examination.

Who do you need in your team?

You might want a team that includes:

GP
Healthcare assistant
Practice nurse
Reception staff
Practice manager
Cleaners.

Table 16.1:   Role and responsibilities checklist – *for each task tick the box for each team member who has a role or responsibility – then note your role and responsibilities for the task*

Completed by: _____

	Primary care team member								What are your roles and your responsibilities?
Task	*Doctor*	*Practice nurse*	*Healthcare assistants*	*Reception team*	*Practice manager*	*Practice secretary*	*Patients*	*Cleaners*	
Identifying those who should be involved in safe-guarding the sharps boxes	✔	✔	✔	✔	✔	✔	✔	✔	*e.g. Making sure that the sharps box is placed out of reach of small children*
Significant event analysis	✔	✔	✔	✔	✔	✔	✔	✔	
Conduct a risk assessment				✔	✔			✔	
Review practice policy		✔	✔	✔	✔	✔			
Develop protocol and related training sessions		✔	✔		✔			✔	

Where you are now

Dr Holiday told the practice manager that she had nearly re-used a contaminated speculum, showing her the neatly (and only just visible) cut opening at the other end of the bag. They completed the first part of the significant event audit form. The practice manager offered to investigate using *Root Cause Analysis* as she had recently learnt about the technique.[1]

What you do next

This might include.

- The practice manager ringing the GP locum who had been filling in for Dr Holiday. This doctor said that she remembered using a speculum on the last day she was there and had put it in the bag on the sink drainer in the room. She was not sure where used equipment should be put. She had looked for a box for used examination equipment on the trolley or the sink unit, but had not seen one and had forgotten to ask about it later.
- The practice manager discussing the incident with all the staff who might have been in Dr Holiday's room while she was away. No one could shed any light on the incident, although the cleaner said that she normally placed any bagged equipment on the trolley, so it was possible she had replaced it, not noticing that it was open. The cleaner said that used instruments were usually left in the sink. She did not think that this was very hygienic, and did not like moving them to the bucket in the treatment room.
- The incident being discussed at a significant event meeting to determine how this type of incident could be avoided. They agreed that:
  - plastic boxes with lids would be placed on each trolley, so that clinicians could place used instruments in them
  - the healthcare assistant (who worked part-time) would collect the boxes and bag the instruments ready for transport to the sterilisation service. She would restock the trolley with clean equipment. The practice nurse would train two of the reception staff to do this when the healthcare assistant was not there
  - the doctors and practice nurses place used equipment in the boxes, not the sink
  - the practice nurse would monitor and oversee the process to reduce risks of cross-infection
  - the incident would be reported as a 'near-miss' via the reporting system set up by the PCO.

What extra resources might this require?

- Purchase of suitably sized plastic boxes with lids.
- The healthcare assistant to start half an hour earlier to deal with used instruments and restock supplies; the receptionists involved need protected time to deputise for this task when the healthcare assistant is not working.
- The receptionists and practice nurse need designated time for training.
- The practice manager needs time to complete the report form for a 'near-miss'.

The outcomes

These might include.

- The risk of re-use of contaminated equipment is avoided.
- Better management of used equipment.
- Prompt restocking of used equipment.
- Avoidance of contamination of other surfaces (sink, etc.) by used equipment, reducing the risk of cross-infection.

How would you demonstrate that you have achieved your outcomes?

The practice nurse, as supervisor of the process, should review the process at three months and then annually to ensure that no problems are arising with the agreed procedure.

Problem case exercise

Problem Case:

Your practice or clinic has a 25-minute power failure that creates havoc. Electronic patient records could not be accessed, prescriptions could not be issued and there was insufficient light to conduct examinations. Patient safety was compromised because recent medical records and medication could not be accessed. How could patients be seen, assessed, diagnosed or treated safely in the situation described?

Who do you need in your team?

Where you are now

Continued

What you do next

What extra resources might this require?

The outcomes

How would you demonstrate that you have achieved your outcomes?

Seven steps to patient safety

More than a million people are treated safely and successfully each year in the NHS but sometimes things go wrong, putting patients at risk. The better your systems are at identifying and managing risk, the safer your practice will be.

The National Patient Safety Agency (NPSA) was set up in 2001 to focus on adverse events and preventing incidents from recurring.[1] Their initial review has resulted in the National Reporting and Learning System (NRLS) being established to assist in:

- identifying trends and patterns of avoidable incidents and underlying causes
- developing and sharing good practice and solutions nationally
- supporting ongoing education and learning.

The seven steps to patient safety described in Box 16.1 provide a practical checklist that can be used to benchmark existing policy and practice by healthcare organisations – trusts or practices, teams or individuals.[1]

Box 16.1:   Seven steps to patient safety[1]

1   *Build a safety culture*: create a culture that is open and fair
2   *Lead and support your staff*: establish a clear and strong focus on patient safety throughout your organisation
3   *Integrate your risk management activity*: develop systems and processes to manage your risks and identify and assess things that could go wrong
4   *Promote reporting*: ensure staff can easily report incidents locally and nationally
5   *Involve and communicate with patients and the public*: develop ways to communicate openly with, and listen to, patients
6   *Learn and share safety lessons*: encourage staff to use root cause analysis to learn how and why incidents happen
7   *Implement solutions to prevent harm*: embed lessons through changes to practice, processes or systems.

You should work through the seven steps, to assess what is currently happening in your trust or practice, and identify the areas that you would like to develop further.

Promoting patient safety

Step 1: Build a safety culture – openness, fairness and integrity

The culture of an organisation simply refers to 'the way things are done around here'. Policies and procedures set out the rules for the workforce to understand and adhere to, but the culture is broader than that. It is also about the boundaries of what is considered to be acceptable or unacceptable ways of behaving by the organisation. Cultures that do not tolerate errors are often referred to as 'blame' cultures, where the emphasis is to punish the guilty rather than learn from errors. Research based in the airline industry shows that the stronger the blame culture, the higher the incident

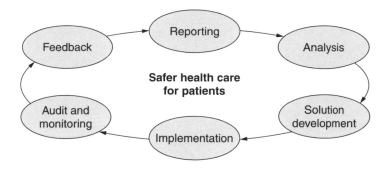

Figure 16.1: Transferring learning into practice.

rate actually is. This is due to a person being reluctant to report 'near misses' or 'serious' incidents because of the consequences of blame being attributed to that individual.

Research into safety in health care has shown that even the best people sometimes make mistakes, and that errors fall into recurrent patterns regardless of the people involved.[2]

If your trust or practice has a supportive learning culture, errors and near misses will be analysed in the interests of improvement. This makes it much easier for staff to report incidents/near misses and prevent poor practice habits from forming.

Continuous quality improvement processes ensure that the trust or practice has a way of transferring learning from regular reviews into professional practice as in Figure 16.1. Use the following.

- Clinical audit to study a particular aspect of a service or condition.
- Service reviews to review all aspects of a service from the viewpoints of clinicians, patients and support workers. Measure the service against the expectations and objectives of the organisation.
- Patient satisfaction surveys to ask patients, carers and the public for their views about a service.
- Staff surveys to ask their views about the organisation and how it operates.
- Quality circles, i.e. a group of people who meet together regularly to identify problems or areas for improvement and work together to implement a solution.

Step 2: Lead and support your staff

Patient safety is everyone's responsibility but building a safer culture depends on strong leadership and commitment from senior managers. They need to acknowledge and act upon messages from the workforce, regardless of their role or level in the organisation (*see* Boxes 16.2, 16.3 and 16.4).

Box 16.2:   What your PCO can do to create a culture that supports learning from adverse incidents

- A Board member has responsibility for patient safety which is viewed as an organisational priority
- Training promotes Health and Safety policies including infection control, medicines management and risk assessment
- Define incidents and near misses
- State clearly what staff need to do when an incident or near miss occurs
- Staff know to whom they should report incidents
- An annual safety assessment survey measures the effectiveness of the reporting and improvement mechanisms
- Identify patient safety ambassadors in each directorate, department or practice who can promote patient safety at every opportunity
- Build patient safety into training programmes and events

Box 16.3:   What you can do to create a culture that supports learning from adverse events in your practice team

- Have a nominated lead for patient safety in your team
- Help the practice team understand the relevance and importance of patient safety and organise appropriate training in the relevant areas
- Staff should feel able to voice their concerns and problems if things go wrong
- Encourage significant event analysis and clinical supervision as reflective tools that identify problems and extract learning from incidents
- Be consistent in applying policies and procedures across your team
- Promote an ethos of openness
- Encourage practice members to challenge assumptions and custom and practice that relate to patient safety in a productive way
- Show that reports received are dealt with fairly and that the appropriate learning and action takes place

Box 16.4:   What you can do to create a culture that supports learning from adverse events as an individual

- Take responsibility for reporting near misses or incidents
- Join in reviews and analyses of situations involving you and your team
- Make necessary changes resulting from an incident review
- Undertake training in relevant areas

Supporting and enabling staff to make patient safety a priority means ensuring that they understand its significance in relation to service delivery and their professional competence. Use the checklist in Box 16.5 to develop your patient safety policy for your practice.

Box 16.5: Checklist for developing a patient safety policy

1   Purpose of the policy
Define why patient safety is important and the standards and indicators that demonstrate good practice
2   Policy context
Refer to other policies or initiatives that affect your patient safety policy
3   Indicators for good practice
  • definition of minimum requirements
  • list of people to whom the standards apply
  • what procedures are followed if standards are not achieved
  • areas where standards can be raised
4   Implementation
  • name of lead person who has main responsibility for monitoring standards
  • list of practical tasks or activities that routinely take place in the application of standards
  • description of the role of patient and public involvement and what mechanisms ensure such involvement takes place
5   Review date for the policy

Step 3: Integrate your risk management activity

Most NHS trusts have robust risk assessment and management policies in place because of their corporate responsibilities for health and safety, clinical governance and user involvement. Your practice needs to make explicit links with and between these policies and programmes. Relate these to the direct actions of your practice team and train them in relevant skills relating to patient safety. Risk management processes include:

  • significant event analysis[3]
  • audit and systematic service reviews[3]
  • clinical supervision.[4,5]

RISK ASSESSMENT
The same process can be adapted for managing all types of risk: financial, managing change, operational, clinical practice and health and safety.

Risk assessment might entail evaluating the risks to the health or well-being or competence of yourself, staff and/or patients in your practice or workplace, and deciding on the action needed to minimise or eliminate those risks.[6]

  • A hazard: something with the potential to cause harm.
  • A risk: the likelihood of that potential to cause harm being realised.

There are five steps to risk assessment.

1   Look for and list the hazards.
2   Decide who might be harmed and how.
3   Evaluate risks arising from the hazards and decide whether existing precautions
    are adequate or more should be done.
4   Record the findings.
5   Review your assessment from time to time and revise it if necessary.

You do not want to spend a lot of time and effort identifying risks or making changes
if they do not matter much. When you have identified a risk, consider:

•   is the risk large?
•   does it happen often?
•   is it a significant risk?

ROOT CAUSE ANALYSIS

Root cause analysis (RCA) is promoted by the National Patient Safety Agency (see its
website).[1] It offers a simple framework in a systematic way gathering and analysing
data that works backwards from the incident and builds up a picture of the environment, people and actions involved (*see* Figure 16.2).

Step 4: Promote reporting

Reporting systems are vital in providing a core of sound, representative information
on which to base your analysis and recommendations.[7] NHS organisations should

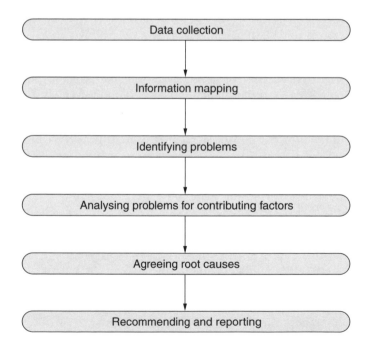

Figure 16.2:   Root cause analysis process.[1]

have (or be developing) a centralised system that gathers data on patient safety incidents. It should cover:

- incidents that have occurred (adverse events or harms)
- incidents that have been prevented (near misses)
- incidents that may happen (risks).

The information can then be used to implement preventative strategies that will protect patients and staff alike as in Boxes 16.6, 16.7 and 16.8. Everyone should be aware of the system and understand how the reporting process works.

Box 16.6: What your PCO can do to promote effective risk management

- Support systematic risk assessment, risk management and incident reporting to be used by the whole workforce
- Include the strategy and action plan for patient safety in the Local Delivery Plan

---

Box 16.7: What your practice team can do to promote effective risk management

- Encourage colleagues to actively report patient safety incidents that happen (including near misses)
- Participate in reviews, audits and reflective practice activities to share good practice and lessons learned

---

Box 16.8: What you can do to promote effective risk management

- Report patient safety incidents that you encounter
- Report risks and hazards that you notice
- Use reflective practice as part of your continuing professional development (CPD) activity and share what you learn with your colleagues

---

Step 5: Involving and communicating with patients and members of the public

Public accountability, transparency and equal access all depend on a degree of user involvement.[8,9] Studies show that patients accept something has gone wrong when they are told about it promptly, fully and compassionately.[10] Involve patients and carers or members of the public in ways that Box 16.9 sets out. Then look at how you can apply this in Boxes 16.10, 16.11 and 16.12.

Box 16.9: Involving patients and the general public

Do	Don't
Include people who have a valid contribution to make	Involve the same people over and over again
Acknowledge and apologise for failings in the care they or their family have received	Ignore or deny genuine concerns or complaints that patients have
Reassure and demonstrate lessons have been learnt from patient safety incidents	Forget to share valuable lessons and to publicise real improvements that result from an incident
Support patients and their families with appropriate systems after involvement in a patient safety incident	Let people try to navigate complex systems without help and signposting

Box 16.10: What your PCO can do to involve and communicate effectively with patients and the public

- Develop a local policy relating to open communication about adverse events with patients
- Ensure that patients are kept fully informed when there has been an incident
- Provide staff with the right education, training and support to enable them to be open and honest with patients and their families

Box 16.11: What your practice team can do to involve and communicate effectively with patients and the public

- Actively involve patients and their families after an incident
- Inform patients and their families if there is a problem, in respectful and sympathetic ways
- Give patients and their families timely information and an apology where it is due

Box 16.12: What you can do to involve and communicate effectively with patients and the public

Further develop your communication skills and be a consistently good communicator

Step 6: Lessons learned

Complaints should be dealt with within the Caldicott framework of confidentiality and accountability.[11] They can be an invaluable source of learning. By looking at the circumstances leading to the event, analysing the event itself and what followed, you can learn what went wrong (if anything did) and consider how it can be prevented from happening again.

The learning needs to be communicated to the rest of the organisation as in Boxes 16.13, 16.14 and 16.15. Use existing mechanisms, such as quality assurance or quality improvement, or performance monitoring. Where learning directly impacts on patient safety, your PCO or practice should recognise and maybe reward good practice. The cost of poor quality is difficult to quantify but the cost of poor patient safety is always too high.

Box 16.13: What PCOs or practices can do to ensure they learn and share safety lessons

- Ensure their staff know about policies and procedures and are trained to undertake appropriate investigations into patient safety incidents
- Describe the criteria of incidents and near misses and define situations when an investigation is needed
- Devise local solutions that can be used when commissioning, redesigning services, for systems improvement and education and training
- Assess the risks and impact of any changes made
- Use good practice identified by other organisations elsewhere in the NHS
- Provide high-quality feedback to staff, the public and patients alike

---

Box 16.14: What your practice team can do to ensure that it learns and shares safety lessons

- Share lessons from its analysis of patient safety incidents within the team
- Share learning with other teams or departments that may be affected by similar issues
- Involve the whole team
- Set up reminders to implement changes consistently
- Give feedback on reported incidents

Box 16.15: What you can do to ensure you learn and share safety lessons

Participate in reflective practice, for example clinical supervision, to identify potential issues and share learning with your colleagues

Step 7: Implement solutions to prevent harm

The action points and solutions should become part of the clinical governance programme within your PCO or practice as in Boxes 16.16, 16.17 and 16.18. The confidence your team has in the process will grow as it sees changes happening.

Box 16.16: What PCOs or practices can do to ensure that they implement solutions to prevent harm

- Look for good practice, or lessons learned, and build up a network to pass on information throughout the workforce
- Reward the actions of individuals and teams that are innovative and consistent in their practice of improving patient safety

---

Box 16.17: What your practice team can do to ensure that it implements solutions to prevent harm

- Use the systems and processes already in place to make changes
- Work with patients and carers to develop solutions
- Build in reminders to promote change consistently within your team

---

Box 16.18: What you can do to ensure that you implement solutions to prevent harm

- Review your practice in order to improve the quality of your performance in a consistent way
- Feed back your experiences to the practice or trust so that others can learn from them

---

Making patient safety a priority takes commitment from the PCO or practice and staff, and consistency from individual practitioners. An increase in reported incidents (initially) means that you are doing things right.

References

1   National Patient Safety Agency (NPSA) (2004) *Introduction to 7 Steps for Patient Safety.* NPSA, London. www.npsa.nhs.uk

2   Reason J (2000) Human error: models and management. *BMJ.* **320**: 768–70.

3   National Institute for Clinical Excellence; Commission for Health Improvement; Royal College of Nursing (2002) *Principles for Best Practice in Clinical Audit.* Radcliffe Medical Press, Oxford.

4   United Kingdom Central Council for Nursing, Midwifery and Health Visiting (1996) *Position Statement on Clinical Supervision for Nursing and Health Visiting.* www. clinical-supervision.com/clinsup.htm

5   University of Manchester (1998) *Clinical Governance and Clinical Supervision: working together to ensure safe and accountable practice.* www.clinical-supervision.com/CG-CS-working.pdf

6   Mohanna K and Chambers R (2000) *Risk Matters in Healthcare.* Radcliffe Medical Press, Oxford.

7   Department of Health (2000) *An Organisation with a Memory.* Department of Health, London.

8   Department of Health (1997) *The New NHS: modern, dependable.* Department of Health, London.

9   Chambers R, Drinkwater C and Boath E (2003) *Involving Patients and the Public* (2e). Radcliffe Medical Press, Oxford.

10   Crane M (2001) What to say if you made a mistake. *Journal of Medical Economics.* **78(16)**: 26–8, 33–4, 36.

11   Department of Health (2003) *Patient Confidentiality and Caldicott Guardians.* Department of Health, London. www.publications.doh.gov.uk/ipu/confiden/

APPENDIX 1

North Staffordshire palliative care communication form

Fax information to: _____

PATIENT DETAILS:

Name:	*Age:*
Address:	*DOB:*
	Sex: M/F

Postcode:

Tel. No:	*Lives alone:* Y/N

CARER DETAILS:

Name:	*Relationship:*
Address:	*Next of kin:* Y/N

Tel. No.:

DIAGNOSIS AND DATE:

Metastases (sites):

Complications:

GP and PRACTICE DETAILS:

Name: Tel. No:

Surgery:

Information:

Palliative care drug pack?	Y/N
Care of the dying pathway?	Y/N
Hospice involved?	Y/N
Hospice at home?	Y/N
Does the coroner need to be informed after death?	Y/N
Is resuscitation information documented in the home?	Y/N
Other relevant information:	

Completed by: _____   **Date:** _____

(PLEASE INFORM OUT-OF-HOURS SERVICE IF THE PATIENT HAS DIED)

APPENDIX 2

Cancer and palliative care: dealing with complex problems in advanced illness

Managing chronic pain in primary care

Not all patients with cancer get pain. Twenty-five per cent of patients will not get significant pain. Of the patients who do get pain, 80% will get more than one pain and 33% will get four or more different pains. Most cancer pain can be managed well by primary care teams.

Support from others can help enormously in some situations. When confronted with a patient in pain it is easy (as a doctor) to feel that the prescription is everything. You cannot do all of these things on your own, involving others early is a good strategy (*see* Box 1 overleaf).

Choosing the right drug

Cancer pains can be managed well if the right drug is given, at the right dose, at the right time. The WHO analgesia ladder in Table 1 is convenient and simple. Table 2 reminds you of the common types of pain you need to be able to treat.

Table 1:   The WHO analgesic ladder

Step	Drug type	Examples
One	Non-opioid +/– adjuvants	Paracetamol
Two	Weak opioid +/– adjuvants	Codeine, Tramadol, Dihydrocodeine
Three	Strong opioid +/– adjuvants	Morphine, Fentanyl, Buprenorphine, Oxycodone

☺ The commonest mistake made is 'not to climb the ladder' but to offer different weak opioids rather than accepting that this patient, at this time, needs to be started on a regular strong opioid.

☺ It is easy to forget that 60 mg of dihydrocodeine six-hourly is approximately equivalent to 5 mg of morphine five times a day – so why not use the morphine? It may cause fewer side-effects and will be effective if the dose is increased.

Box 1:   Pain management strategy

Taking a history	Sort the pain(s) out in your head. Reflect back what the patient is saying to you 'let me see if I have this right ... the pain in your arm started as a burning discomfort a week ago ...'. This ensures you have the story and demonstrates you are listening (which helps to unwind anxiety and fear which have been making the pain worse ...).
Examination	Confirms trust. Helps to elucidate likely causes for each pain.
Explanation	Start from what the patient knows 'What do you think is causing this pain?'. Get a feel for how much the patient wants to know. Use simple language and be prepared to say the same thing several times (diagrams can help). Uncertainty provokes anxiety that provokes more pain. Acknowledge concerns and avoid inappropriate reassurance. 'Everything's going to be alright' is probably a useless lie. 'Over the next two days we will work on getting your pain controlled so that you can be comfortable sitting down' is realistic, and for the patient a genuine source of hope.
Elevation of pain threshold	Prescribed drugs: analgesics, antidepressants and anxiolytics. What are the things causing most distress for the patient? They may not be anything you can influence but others may be able to help (such as social or psychological factors or spiritual pain).
Lifestyle modification	Consider whether pain provoking activities can be done differently? Can a painful limb be supported? Can the environment be changed through aids or adaptations to reduce the impact of painful activity? You may not know the answer so involve the district nursing team, physiotherapists or local authority occupational therapists for an assessment.
Modification of the pathological process	Radiotherapy works for more than 80% of those with metastatic bone pain as well as for nerve compression syndromes. It takes about two weeks to be effective. If the patient is likely to survive longer than that it is always worth discussing the option with a member of the oncology team. Even in advanced cancers chemotherapy or hormone manipulation can sometimes be very useful as 'add on' analgesia. Carcinoma of the prostate is a good example of the latter. Orthopaedic surgery has an important role in management of existing or potential pathological fractures of long bones.
Interruption of pain pathways	Peripheral and epidural nerve blocks are needed infrequently but are the 'only thing that works' in some situations. The anaesthetic department or hospice consultant staff can give advice about this. If in doubt ask!

Table 2: Treatment of common types of pain

Quality of pain	Timing	Aggravating and relieving factors	Radiation	Type of pain	Notes on analgesia
Aching, poorly localised	Continuous, gradual onset and increasing severity	Local heat (relieves)		**Visceral**	Opiate-sensitive. Gastritis best treated with proton pump inhibitor drug
Aching, soreness – some localisation and tenderness				**Soft tissue inflammation**	
Sharp gripping, severe cramp	Sudden onset and intermittent but repetitive			**Smooth muscle spasm, e.g. bowel colic**	Can be opiate-sensitive. Can try antispasmodics orally or subcutaneously
Aching, soreness, well localised, local tenderness	Intermittent or constant, gradual onset and increasing in severity	Movement and weight bearing or direct pressure. Eased with rest or posture change		**Bone pain**	Can be partially opiate-sensitive. NSAID useful. Consider radiotherapy
Aching, throbbing, burning, stinging, numbness, reduced or altered sensation, allodynia	Constant	Touch (worsens)	Peripheral lesions can follow dermatone	**Neuropathic pain Nerve compression and/or nerve damage/injury**	Can be opiate-sensitive. Difficult pains to relieve (seek advice). Dexamethasone, amitriptyline, gabapentin and others have been used
Sharp, shooting, stabbing, lancinating	Intermittent, spontaneous	Movement (worsens)			
Sharp chest wall – pain on inspiration	Intermittent	Coughing (worsens)		**Pleuritic pain**	Opiate-sensitive. NSAID also useful. More difficult if co-existent thoracic nerve infiltration

Continued

Table 2: *Continued*

Quality of pain	Timing	Aggravating and relieving factors	Radiation	Type of pain	Notes on analgesia
Sharp pain right subcostal margin and right hypochondrium	Intermittent	Movement inspiration – local pressure		**Liver capsule distension pain**	Opiate-sensitive. Steroids also useful
Aching/soreness radiating 'non-dermatomally' usually around neck, shoulder, hip girdle, lumbar spine; with local muscular tender spots	Worse after rest	Anxiety worsens. Physiotherapy, local heat, stretching or acupuncture reduce		**Myofascial pain**	Not opiate-sensitive, usually arise from cancer-related disability
Gradual onset superficial burning and deep ache, reduced or altered sensation trophic changes, muscle wasting and fatigue	Intermittent or constant	Worse with deep pressure	Sympathetic nerve distribution (mirrors arterial supply)	**Sympathetic mediated pain (uncommon, but difficult to control)**	Can try as neuropathic pain above

Adapted and reproduced by permission of Dr G Barkby, St Catherine's Hospice, Preston

Considering morphine as the next analgesic

This is **strongly recommended** if:

- your patient has one or more pains that are poorly controlled with 60 mg codeine six-hourly (or equivalent)
- your patient's pain is not better managed with a more specific treatment (e.g. relieving constipation, proton-pump inhibitor for gastritis, antispasmodic for simple gut colic)
- your patient has a pain that is likely to be sensitive to morphine. If a patient gets partial relief from regular codeine (four to six-hourly) then it is likely that they do! In practice, the only way to know is to try.

WHAT DO YOU DO FIRST?

Explain to your patient that you would like to start them on a more effective treatment for their pain and that:

1 the dose needed varies between people
2 the first goal is a reduction in discomfort so that sleep is possible
3 the common side-effects are sleepiness, nausea and constipation. Drowsiness will wear off after a few days, but you are going to provide them with some treatment to minimise problems from nausea and constipation.

START WITH ORAL MORPHINE MIXTURE 2 MG/ML (10 MG IN FIVE ML SPOONFUL)

- Suggest they take one 5 ml spoonful (10 mg) *every* four hours whilst they are awake, unless they are very frail or elderly (use 5 mg) or already on an alternative strong opiate (in this case you will need to calculate a dose equivalent so as not to under-dose the patient).
- If this dose does not provide any relief at all then increase the dose by 50% and repeat after two hours.
- If this dose provides some relief but the effect wears off before four hours, they should increase the dose by 50%, take the next dose early and continue at the higher dose at four-hourly intervals.
- A night time dose can be twice the standard day time dose (1.5 times for very frail or elderly).
- Frequency and dose should be recorded by the patient so that 24-hour requirements can be calculated.
- If the patient has no need for an anti-emetic then prescribe haloperidol 1.5 mg with the first dose of morphine and continue 1.5 to 3 mg at night. Metoclopramide 10 mg three times daily is an alternative.
- A stimulant laxative is very likely to be needed. Co-danthrusate (2 tablets) at night is a sensible start.

Review

Review the patient soon. There are always anxieties about starting morphine which need to be explored. Commonly, patients are hesitant about taking repeated four-hourly doses if they are in less or no pain. Fear of dependence or of the drug 'not working' later in the illness is also commonly expressed. Reassurance *is* appropriate for both of these issues!

If the patient's pain(s) is now controlled

- Work out how much morphine has been used over the last 24 hours.
- Prescribe this as half the total twice daily using a slow release morphine preparation.
- The controlled release tablet can be given instead of a four-hourly dose – the previous advice to give both together is probably unnecessary.
- 'Breakthrough' pain should be managed using morphine mixture or immediate release morphine tablets (do not confuse these with slow release preparations). The correct dose is the equivalent four-hourly dose. (For example, if a patient is taking 60 mg MST twice daily [bd], this is equivalent to 120 mg of morphine per day and the correct breakthrough dose would be 20 mg [10 ml of morphine 10 mg/5 ml].)
- The total dose of breakthrough medication used in a 24-hour period should be added to the slow release dosage given on the following day.
- The anti-emetic drug can often be stopped after a week.
- The laxative almost always needs to be continued.

If the patient's pains are not controlled

- Is the drug being taken and absorbed (ask again about vomiting)?
- Are you being realistic? It can take three to five or more days to titrate the dose so that the patient is comfortable at rest. Pain free movement is often more difficult to achieve.
- Review the pain management options lists in Tables 1 and 2. Try adjuvant analgesia.
- Inflammatory conditions and especially bone pain can be relieved with NSAIDs such as naproxen 500 mg bd.
- If the pain has a neuropathic quality (burning or stabbing pain, often with a background of reduced sensation) try these in turn: add amitriptyline 10–25 mg at night and increase to 75 mg (take care in the elderly); substitute gabapentin for amitriptyline, 300 mg initially then increasing by 300 mg daily up to 600 mg three times daily; add dexamethasone 8 mg in the morning. (This will sometimes convert neuropathic pain into a more morphine sensitive pain.)
- Consider the need for anxiolytics such as diazepam 2–5 mg or antidepressants.
- Consider the possibility of hypercalcaemia (rarely identified in the primary care setting but can occur in up to 10% of cases of advanced malignancy – a high index of suspicion is required).
- Do not be afraid of asking for help. Difficult pains can be very difficult indeed!

Managing the terminal phase

The Macmillan Gold Standards[1] and the Liverpool Marie Curie integrated care pathway for the dying[2] provide very clear descriptions of what high-quality care should look like. In brief, impending death can be recognised in those with advanced malignancy by the patient being:

- bedbound: with profound weakness, requiring assistance with all care
- semi-comatose: drowsy with reduced cognition (though may have very lucid moments)

- only able to take sips of fluids
- no longer able to take tablets.

It is sensible to seek agreement from the team that a patient has entered the terminal phase of their illness.

Common concerns for patients in the terminal phase

- Death itself.
- The process of dying.
- Grief over the sequential loss that he or she has already suffered.
- Past experiences.
- Worries over current treatment.
- Anguish or spiritual distress.

The clinical team should review the patient and plan how to manage any worsening of symptoms

The symptoms are:

- pain (often more than one)
- dyspnoea and/or noisy breathing
- nausea/vomiting
- confusion
- agitation
- urinary incontinence/retention
- dry, sore mouth.

Review the needs of non-professional carers too

- They have to function in other ways – at work themselves and/or as parents.
- Exhaustion of a 24/7 job!
- Anticipate intercurrent illness which is extremely common especially in older spouses.
- Acknowledge their great uncertainty – which is confidence eroding.
- Obtain practical help (night time support is particularly important).
- Get appropriate aids.
- Be sensitive to role conflicts that arise (e.g. daughter providing personal care for her father).

Ensure that carers have had time to ventilate concerns – this is critical because if you can reduce the uncertainties for the family you will reduce their anxiety. Rising anxiety often precipitates emergency transfer of the patient to hospital during a terminal illness. Common fears and worries are:

- that the patient is not eating/drinking
- that the patient is not taking medication
- that the process of dying will be in some way horrific
- the nature of help they can expect and from whom
- who to contact in an emergency and how
- what the possible problems are (and what is the plan for dealing with them)
- recognising that death has occurred
- knowing what to do after death.

Managing the five common symptoms

Anticipate that each of these might occur and issue a prescription and written instructions for the management of each when you decide that a patient has entered the terminal stage of their illness. The five common symptoms are as follows.

* Pain
* Nausea and vomiting
* Respiratory tract secretions
* Agitation
* Dyspnoea.

Pain

If the patient has no pain anticipate that it might occur:

* prescribe diamorphine 2.5 mg as a required dose
* remember water for injection with written instructions if nursing staff coming in to see a patient are to be effective.

If the patient has pain but has not been taking any strong analgesia:

* prescribe 2.5–5 mg diamorphine as a stat dose
* start diamorphine 10 mg–30 mg via syringe driver
* prescribe 'as required' additional doses of diamorphine as a sixth of the 24-hour dose
* add an anti-emetic to the syringe driver.

If the patient's pain was controlled by taking oral morphine or other strong opioid:

* prescribe diamorphine via syringe driver using the 24-hour total dose of oral morphine divided by three (for example, 60 mg MST twice daily would require 40 mg of diamorphine over 24 hours)
* prescribe as required diamorphine subcutaneously (s/c) i.e. 24-hour dose of diamorphine divided by six.

If the patient's pain is not controlled increase the analgesia dose by 33% as the driver is started.

Nausea and vomiting

If a patient does not have nausea or vomiting then anticipate that this might occur:

* prescribe cyclizine 50 mg s/c as a required dose
* provide a written instruction for appropriate use.

If nausea and/or vomiting are present:

* prescribe cyclizine 50 mg s/c as a stat dose
* prescribe cyclizine 150 mg s/c via syringe driver.

Agitation

If agitation is not present then anticipate that it might occur:

* prescribe midazolam 2.5–5 mg s/c as a required (prn) dose
* provide a written instruction for its appropriate use.

If the patient is already becoming restless or agitated:

- prescribe midazolam 2.5–5 mg s/c as a stat dose
- prescribe 10–60 mg s/c via syringe driver (usual starting dose 20 mg)
- prescribe 2.5–5 mg midazolam s/c as a prn dose.

Respiratory tract secretions (rattling breathing)

If breathing is quiet anticipate that secretions may build up:

- prescribe glycopyrronium 0.2 mg s/c as a prn dose
- provide a written instruction for appropriate use.

If respiratory tract secretions are building up and the patient is developing noisy breathing:

- prescribe glycopyrronium 0.2 mg s/c as a stat dose
- prescribe glycopyrronium 0.6–1.2 mg via syringe driver
- prescribe glycopyrronium 0.2 mg s/c prn.

Dyspnoea

If dyspnoea is not present anticipate that it might occur:

- prescribe diamorphine 2.5–5 mg s/c as a prn dose
- make it clear that an appropriately calculated additional dose of diamorphine can be used if the patient is already taking diamorphine as an analgesic. This can be the same one-sixth daily dose as used for breakthrough pain
- provide written instructions for appropriate use.

If dyspnoea is present:

- give explanation and companionship
- fan/open window
- consider oxygen
- nebulised bronchodilators for bronchospasm
- diuretics for heart failure.

If dyspnoea is still present administer an appropriate (one-sixth of the total daily) prn diamorphine dose and be prepared to increase the total daily dose accordingly. If the patient is not taking diamorphine:

- prescribe diamorphine 2.5–5 mg s/c as a stat and prn dose
- prescribe diamorphine 10–30 mg s/c via syringe driver
- provide written instructions for appropriate use.

References

1   Useful information about the *Gold Standards Framework* from the Macmillan Site www.macmillan.org.uk/healthprofessionals/disppage.asp?id=6875

2   Useful information about the *Liverpool Care Pathway for the dying patient* can be found at www.lcp-mariecurie.org.uk/ – examples of the pathway are downloadable in pdf.

Index